D1489594

# SECOND SPRING

# Mel London
# SECOND SPRING

## You Can Make
## The Middle Years
## The Best Years
## Of Your Life –

### And Don't Believe
### Anyone Who Tells
### You Different!

Rodale Press, Emmaus, Pa.

Book design by Linda Jacopetti

Printed in the United States of America on recycled paper containing a high percentage of de-inked fiber.

**Library of Congress Cataloging in Publication Data**

London, Mel.
    Second spring.

    Includes index.
    1. Middle age.  2. Aging.  3. Conflict of generations.
I. Title
HQ1059.4.L66              305.2′44              82-3855
ISBN 0-87857-397-6   hardcover              AACR2


2   4   6   8   10   9   7   5   3        hardcover

*For all my old friends*
*who are younger than springtime:*

Flora, Seymour, George, Jackie, Rudy and Carol, Lewis, Carmen and Helena, Malcolm, Eve, Uncle John, Mike and Debbie, Gerry and Gloria, Dina and Alex, Dorrie and Joel, and especially Joe Longo.

# Contents

# Acknowledgments

Some years back, during the euphoria that accompanies seeing a first book in print, I made the disconcerting discovery that I had left out the name of a man who had been so very valuable to me during the pregnancy period of trying to fill the empty pages. It has created a minor paranoia that stays with me until this very day as I attack the pleasant chore of listing the people who have been both invaluable and supportive in the year of writing this book. I have tried to mention each and every one who has provided that special degree of encouragement and knowledge, without which I could not have completed the journey. I hope I have omitted no one this time.

We are, all of us, influenced in no small measure by the ideas of others, through a special "chemistry" that tells us that there is a freshness of thinking, a breaking of the bonds of the stultifying past, in the words that they speak and write. The thinking of Dr. Bernice Neugarten and the advocacy of Maggie Kuhn fall so well into that category, and I have been influenced greatly by them. I am, at this point, an ardent admirer of both. My thanks also go to Dr. Robert Mendelsohn, Dr. Stephen Z. Cohen, and Marty Knowlton; to Dr. Richard Gruelich and Daniel Rogers of the Gerontology Research Center; to Dr. Richard H. Davis of the Andrus Gerontology Center; and to Dr.

Manny Riklan and Janet Beard at St. Barnabas Hospital for their support and their invaluable and provocative information, much of which appears in the chapters that follow.

U.S. Representative Geraldine Ferraro was one of the first to make me aware of the distortions taking place in the projections for the Social Security system and it was through her that I found Robert M. Ball. I am grateful to both of them for helping to balance the discussion. My thanks, too, for the help from The Older Women's League—especially to Dr. Ruby Benjamin and Jean Phillips—and to the Displaced Homemakers' Network, to Elderhostel and Michael Zoob, and to Barbara Hertz and Roberta Gerry of *Prime Time* magazine. Dr. George Gerbner and his staff at the Annenberg School, University of Pennsylvania, made a superb contribution with their reporting and analyses of the media. Thanks to Tom Walker and Nina Kenny at Colonial Penn Group, to Dr. James C. Hall of Pace University, and to Dr. Jim Gallagher of Career Management Associates for their help in the areas of education and career-changing. I would also like to thank Anne Luck for her help in the research phase of the book, and Ralph Bowers and Irene Levitt of NRTA/AARP for their help and early encouragement in the development of the subject matter that would fill the pages.

The staff of Rodale Press has now been with me through so many books that they already know the words I use too often, the grammatical mistakes I stumble over (over which I stumble?), and the peculiarities of my ancient typewriter. To Camille Bucci of Rodale who kept track of changes in this manuscript, without missing a comma or misplacing an insert, my thanks for her ever-ready assistance.

And for Charles Gerras, my editor, who always seems to be last in these listings, my recognition for having the patience of a saint and the humor that makes me feel well loved through the ordeal of one year of writing. To him—and to all the others—listed and unlisted—remembered and inadvertently omitted—my deepest thanks for making this journey so memorable.

Mel London
Fire Island, N.Y.

# A Sometimes Humorous Often Serious Very Necessary Introduction

## I.

It was bound to happen to me. It had never happened before, though I am certain that, in the deep, dark recesses of my mind, it was a possibility that had been pushed even deeper each time it threatened to surface. It was a first time, and I'm sure the look on my face gave away all the hidden feelings, the twist of anguish and distress mingled with the awful need to laugh aloud. It was obviously important to me, terribly, terribly important, or I would not have chosen it to open this book.

We were on the Third Avenue bus in New York, and it was a brilliant Saturday afternoon, filled with the promise of the vitality "uptown" and pre-Christmas shopping, the hum of kinetic energy that so characterizes every shopping area before the holidays. The bus, empty when we began our trip, soon became filled with bundled-up wintertime passengers, all of them bound for the department stores.

An elderly lady got on, making her way falteringly past the driver as she paid her fare, and I rose to give her my seat. She smiled at me, sat down, and I turned to move away. A young man, about 25, then rose, nodded slightly, *and offered me his seat!*

Of course, I was startled. For an instant I refused to realize that it was I to whom he was nodding. I am an active filmmaker and you must understand that there is no doubt in my mind that I could outlast that young man on an extended film trip through the world. I could carry more equipment and be less tired than he would be while working at an altitude of 14,000 feet in Bolivia. I could survive more easily in the funk of a jungle or the aridly oppressive heat of a desert, work longer hours, function efficiently with less sleep, and then offer *him my* seat on a bus were he to get aboard last!

But that is not the point, is it? Arriving home, I looked carefully in the mirror. Undoubtedly, to that young man I looked middle-aged, at least; possibly he saw in me the early stages of a gerontological disintegration. Belatedly, I appreciated his kind and thoughtful gesture.

A short time later, while reading Malcolm Cowley's delightful minibook *The View from 80* (Viking Press, New York, 1980), I laughed when I came across his own description of just such an occurrence. It was on the Madison Avenue bus in his case, and it obviously made as strong an impression upon him as it had on me.

And so it comes to us in a variety of ways, for each of us at a different time in what we have begun to call our "middle lives." Possibly it happens when the children leave home, or when a reassessment of a career becomes a vital emotional enigma. It is, whatever the personal catalyst, a realization that for some time we have been looking at middle age from the opposite side of the calendar. Whether on a bus, or by some chance remark, or by a stroke of inner genius, we suddenly realize, as the cartoon character Pogo might have said, "Them is us!" But as this book took shape I found, to my surprise, that the norm was not a *negative* feeling about reaching middle age, but a very positive view of what we *are* rather than what we *were,* and a reassessment that occurs for the express purpose of determining *what it is we want to be* during these coming generations of our lives.

In setting the parameters I decided to look carefully at the generation between the ages of 45 and 65, hoping that people under the limit would read the book because they will eventually join us, and hoping just as strongly that everyone over the limit would also read it, for some of the most dynamic personalities in my research were between the ages of 65 and 85! But in narrowing the research to the 20 years between 45 and 65 I discovered some remarkable things about us— and, therefore, about myself.

Our generation is, in fact, the most active, most affluent, and in many respects, the strongest group in American society, but you'd never know it from reading what's around. We've reached a stage where we have more freedom than we've ever had, and though we represent only one-quarter of the population (and we're growing), we earn 50 percent of the income in the country. Career-changing is a dynamic part of the life style of those of us who have passed the age of 45 and it is much more prevalent than people think. More and more of our age group are going back to college either full-time for degree courses or part-time for myriad personal reasons. The health problems of our generation are terribly overemphasized. The myths of the "empty-nest syndrome" and "midlife crisis" are bandied about, but, essentially, both are fallacies of our current societal thinking.

Of course, we are changing. When have we not? At what point in our lives did we not face change and the need for response to that change? For some reason, however, as we reach midlife, the word "change" seems to give way to the word "crisis" and society demands that we think differently about ourselves as we reach whatever magic age is decreed to be a "crisis" point. And we, gentle sheep that we are, begin to accept what society wants us to believe—that it is time to move aside and leave the harvest to the young. We can no longer accept that.

And so this is a book that not only speaks of change as it affects us. It is a book of observation, a book of euphoria at having reached an age where we can no longer be put into neat categories, rigid "stages" of life; where we are discovering that our age group is more confident, more adventurous, more interesting, more eager to enjoy the fruits of our labor, and more filled with a sense of growth than ever before in our lives. It is also, in its own way, a book that reflects my anger and distress at the inequity of a lack of social recognition for an entire segment of our population. And I am not alone, for I have begun to hear this anger all around me. New groups and new voices are rising irately against the unfairness that relegates almost half of America to a pasture of distortion and myth—unobserved, unnoticed, unheard.

# II.

I am not, by any means, a Pollyanna. My first interest in the subject of aging dates back more than 20 years, when I was involved in a series of films that took me to chronic disease hospitals, nursing homes, and facilities for the aged blind and deaf. I have seen enough pain and suffering to last a lifetime, and that is perhaps another reason that I have decided to write a book about the aging process, one that looks more optimistically at where we are in life and opens new avenues of discovery at this most exciting time.

I watched for five slow, agonizing years as my wife ministered to her own mother through senility, disease, and the wasting away of the body and senses. During the writing of this book my sister-in-law died at the age of 60 after a debilitating and horrifying battle with cancer. My Academy Award nomination for best documentary film was for a film on the subject of Parkinson's disease and aging (1963: *To Live Again*). I am only too aware of just how vulnerable we are and I, like you, have watched close friends succumb to a variety of diseases, all the while hearing that we live longer now (and we do).

Problems? Of course there are problems. But that is exactly the point. At what time in your life did they *not* occur? If problems are the private domain of the aging, why is the suicide rate so high among teen-agers and young adults? Too much of what has been written or said about us has been spelled out by "experts" who are much younger than we are. At a conference on aging held in Iowa last year, a discussion leader of about 30 was summing up some suggestions when a feisty, gray-haired older woman stood up and shouted, "I came to Des Moines to hear older women speak. I'm getting tired of having all you younger women telling me what my problems are, and patronizing me. How can you know what it's like to be old?"

And so I, who am not a sociologist, psychologist, psychiatrist, gerontologist, social worker, or medical doctor, ask you to share this personal journey with me, for it has taken me all my 57 years to "research" what follows on these pages. I changed my career at the age of 57, the year in which this book is being written. I found, to my surprise, that many of my friends were contemplating just such a change, and some were much older than I. My friend Carmen bought an old, burned-out, stone house in upstate New York, and he is reconstructing it, stone by stone, by himself, whenever he can spare the time. The fact that Carmen is 60 and an active filmmaker, sculptor, painter, animator, and ham radio operator, plus the fact that it will take him at least 40 more years to complete the construction job, does not faze him in the least. Most of all, for Carmen, there is time. Best of all, there is his attitude.

Through it all, possibly you will discover several things with me. We will not meet anyone who is getting younger. But there are distinct advantages to getting older. Most important of all, you will find—as I have—that the archaic theory of "life stages" is fast losing support. I am, give or take ten years or so, about your age. It becomes my prerogative, then, to ask you to share this most personal journey with me.

# III.

It is winter on Fire Island as I begin. The village is once again empty and, when the wind blows from the south, I can hear the hushed roar of the ocean just a few yards away. Perhaps it is an omen, but each time I have begun a book here, one of the winter deer has appeared on the dunes. A few moments ago a large buck crested the horizon, stood for an instant atop the dune, and then disappeared toward the sea. Snow is forecast for this evening and I look forward to the first drifts that will appear on our walk tomorrow morning in a breathless beauty of white, dusty powder. The pines will carry a mantle of crystalline snow and I shall have to awaken early to shake their branches and relieve them of their burden. As I sit here I think with delight of a story that was told to me by my friend Lewis Freedman.

George Santayana was invited to speak to the student body of Harvard University. It was early April a long, long time ago. The students, about 300 of them, had assembled in the large, ramped lecture hall when Santayana entered and walked to the podium. He paused, looked around the hall, and then glanced out the window near the lectern. There, brilliant in their yellow glory, the forsythia had begun to bloom. Santayana looked again at the students, all of them waiting to hear what the great man would say. "Excuse me, gentlemen," he said with a smile. "I have a date with Spring." And he walked out of the lecture hall and into the garden.

And I, too, have a date with Spring—for the second time.

# Part I
# The Invisible Generations

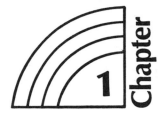

# The Great American Disappearing Act

> *When you get there, there is no there there.*
> *Gertrude Stein*

As a child I was a great movie fan. Saturday morning was the beginning of an all-day odyssey that took me through 3 features, 14 short subjects, a Flash Gordon (or Buck Rogers or Tarzan) serial, 4 games of Kid-Bingo or Keeno or Banko, plus door prizes of bicycles, Monopoly sets, or roller skates (none of which I ever won). All for ten cents! My only sustenance was a large bag of jelly beans, purchased for another five cents at the local Woolworth's, and by seven o'clock that evening, my mother might have the police out looking for the wayward son who had not yet returned from an "afternoon" at the movies at the Park Plaza Theater, only two blocks away.

So many years later, as a filmmaker, I think back to the motion pictures that still stay with me, and there are many that come to mind. Fredric March and his miraculous and spine-chilling transformation from Dr. Jekyll to Mr. Hyde. Lon Chaney as the original and unsurpassed Phantom of the Opera. My first loves and childhood passions:  3

Fay Wray and Helen Twelvetrees. Above all, the "movie magic" of Claude Rains in *The Invisible Man*.

In glorious black and white and with scratchy sound, this film portrayed a figure bandaged to the top of his head, only the sculptured shape of the gauze indicating that there was a human face underneath. I remember sitting breathlessly as he unwound the strands of the bandage slowly, deliberately, revealing that under it all there was—nothing! He had disappeared, for beneath the bandage no flesh could be seen. He strode undetected through the real world, the only clue to his existence being the footprints he left in the snow.

During the intense and exciting year in which I researched this book, it all came back to me vividly and with a sense of impotent anguish. When we are children, adolescents, or young adults, the behavioral scientists study, analyze, and dissect us. They interpret everything we do or say or think, and even some of the things we never thought. Our rebellions are evaluated as normal and then reevaluated as abnormal if we go too far.

As we grow, go out into the world of business, marry or develop a relationship with someone else, or possibly have children and then send them on their way, the writers find it quite easy to categorize us and put us into little compartments. Sometime after the of 40, we seem to stabilize for the researchers and they skip a generation, suddenly to discover us again at 65.

Unfortunately, 65 is a mystical, burdensome number that was forced upon us by legislative history. There is no other reason for it. Back in the '30s, when Congress had to find an age for retirement and Social Security, 65 seemed a logical place to begin (or end?). The fact that the society was different at that time, that we were in the midst of a terrible economic depression, does not seem to have changed things through the years. Even today the scientists, sociologists, physicians, and philosophers pick us up again at 65 for a microscopic study of our emotional needs, our physical disintegration, our financial status, our sexual nonrequirements, our nutritional poverty, and our rapid slide into senility. The fact that most studies in the past have concentrated on the *needy* aged seems to have had no real impact on the thinking of our society. Though only 5 percent of all people over 65 are in rest homes or nursing homes, while the remainder live comfortably and vitally within their communities, the myths of fragility and invalidism that have sprung up about the aging persist.

What, then, about the years in between? What happens to the

age group between 40 or 45 and 65? What happens to *us*, those of us who feel that between those two ages we barely seem to exist? Through all the papers, the books, the monographs, the scientific studies, the surveys, and the magazine articles, we begin to feel as Claude Rains must have felt. We are there under all those bandages of experience, but no one seems to see us for 20 whole years—*nearly a full generation!* Sometimes we get the feeling that we haven't even left our tracks in the snow. To put the thing another way, we are groundhogs who come up to see if our shadows are visible at the age of 45 and, seeing nothing, we descend again under the forest floor, to reappear at 65.

The more perceptive researchers, such as Dr. Bernice Neugarten of the University of Chicago, have also discovered this strange disappearance of millions of people. She has written that the years of maturity are, indeed, much less understood than those of the early life experiences or the years that follow the onset of old age. Somehow the scientists assume that all the decisions of any importance, all the significant events, all the emotional traumas (with the exception of "midlife crisis," which I shall cover later) have already been lived. Obviously, nothing ever happens between the ages of 40 and 65!

In our daily lives the phenomenon continues and, especially for women, our generation is almost totally invisible. All our vitality, all our financial strength as consumers, all our achievements are barely touched on in the media (especially television and advertising) or in popular literature.

Several years ago Gail Sheehy wrote her best-selling study on "Predictable Crises of Adult Life" in *Passages* (Bantam, New York, 1977), in which she covered 115 case histories of people in midlife. In 514 pages (a very thick book by any standards) she devoted *only 19* of them to people over 45 years of age! In those final pages one slight mention is made of someone over 55, but other than that, we do not exist in her book. We simply are not there and all our "predictable crises" have already occurred. A friend of mine, interviewed by me for *Second Spring* angrily told me, "I was furious. I've just turned 50 and I couldn't find myself in her book." Possibly it is because Sheehy defines "midlife" as the middle 30s!

In still another best-seller, *The Seasons of a Man's Life* (Ballantine, New York, 1978), Daniel Levinson presupposes early in his preface that every middle-aged person is negative toward that stage in life. I thought it would be a turnoff for me but I must admit that I enjoyed Levinson's book a great deal more than Sheehy's popular reportage.

Nevertheless, his study is based upon only *40 men* (with women re-maining invisible again, this time since Levinson had limited funding and felt that it was better to study 40 men in depth than to divide the sexes at 20 apiece). All his subjects were from the Northeast and all were in one of four categories: biologists, novelists, executives, or blue collar workers. The rest of us are to assume that our "midlife" times are reflective of his subjects, no matter what our backgrounds, our jobs, our economic status, or our geographic location.

More important, perhaps, and more germane to my feelings of invisibility, is the fact that Levinson also stops at the other side of the dividing line, and in his period of "middle adulthood" age 45 to 60 is not touched upon at all! We are passed off—the millions of us—with the statement that our bodily powers and our mental faculties will somewhat diminish after the age of 40. But then he goes on to state that many of humanity's most ingenious and brilliant achievements take place during those invisible years—in science, the arts, teaching, business, politics, international diplomacy, and philosophy. Indeed, as I read it, I could not for the life of me remember a brilliant philosopher who was *18* years of age!

Even in the more scientific surveys we are either "lumped" or "bumped." One of the best of these studies was conducted by Louis Harris Associates for the National Council on the Aging in 1975. It analyzes public attitudes on aging and it is titled *The Myth and Reality of Aging in America.* I will refer to many of its findings in later chapters, but I was again struck by an interesting phenomenon. Over 4,000 in-person household interviews were done during the late spring and early summer of 1974. There were two basic groups of interviewees: the general public and those over 65, the former including everyone be-tween the ages of 18 and 64! Somehow it became uncomfortable to think that I had exactly the same feelings about something as important as aging as did my young friends of 18 or 20 or 30.

The surveys that are conducted on "adult" education do very much the same thing, and everyone over the age of 25 is considered an adult student!

The final point I'd like to make has nothing at all to do with our invisibility, but rather with the tendency of Americans to put everything and everyone into neat, gift-wrapped packages. I get the feeling that if we don't fit into a category, we somehow are discarded to keep the statistics tidy and uncluttered. In all the literature that I read while doing the research for this book (with a few outstanding exceptions, such as the work by Dr. Neugarten), the tendency to put everyone into stages, transitions, passages, and life straitjackets began to upset me, for the more I read and the more people I spoke to, the more I realized that there is no average American, young or old—or middle-aged.

The society, and thus the demography of the aging, have changed so rapidly in the past 20 years that it is well-nigh impossible to state that we can be put into a specific category at a certain age. In fact, I sincerely doubt that there ever was such a time.

Other surveys and popular books concern themselves only with the middle-class heterosexual combinations. It is easier to show how children affect the growth or stagnation of a marriage than it is to discuss childless marriages or people who have never married at all. The entrance into middle life (whatever the chronological age) seems not to distinguish among sexual preference, marital status, and the sex of the subjects themselves. If the man of our generation thinks he is invisible, the woman must be even angrier and more frustrated. One well-known study (by Dr. George Vaillant), for example, covers the lives of only 95 men—*all Harvard graduates!* It is no wonder that some of us feel that we have been assembly-lined as people, expected to perform the necessary changes as each age comes upon us.

It may be just a coincidence, but, ever since that young man got up and offered me his seat on the bus, I have been doing a lot more walking! The other day I was strolling uptown on my way to an appointment and I noticed the signs in the windows of the savings banks. Right along with the weekly rates for six-month certificates of deposit, the bold, red signs in the windows proclaimed: NEW LOW RATES FOR SAVINGS BANK LIFE INSURANCE. INQUIRE WITHIN! I read on to find that there were new, lower rates on five-year renewable term policies and that the annual premium had been slashed (also in capital letters). Of course, since women live longer than men, their rates were even lower. I quickly skimmed the ages, past 20, 25, 30, 35, 40—and then it stopped, right at 45! No more. Ended. Finished. The bargain is sealed, but only up to 45. I looked in vain to see if, perhaps, they had slashed my rates, too. Nothing. Nothing older than 45. Of course, they had figures for me inside the bank. But no more bargains. Certainly not at 57.

Once again I felt invisible. Or, at least, shoved into the closet until I reached 65, when they might again discover me.

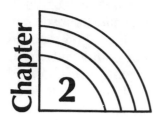

2

# "Excuse Me, Sir (or Madam), Could You Direct Me to Middle Age?"

> Middle age is when you're faced with two temp-
> tations and you choose the one that will get you
> home by nine o'clock.
>
> Pres. Ronald Reagan

I've used the quote by President Reagan not because I think it's true but because I think it's typical. Long the butt of jokes, long reflective of the stereotypes and myths you will read about in the next chapter, middle age is actually impossible to define. At least it is absurd to try to categorize it at all in this generation. But that doesn't seem to stop anyone from trying.

For example, think for a moment and then give your definition of "middle age." Is it a chronological description? A personal, emotional one? A textbook definition? If you succeed on the first one, try giving a definition of "old age." Easier? Not for most. It just depends upon which side of the fulcrum you swing from.

If you listen, if you read, if you watch television, if you are 30 or 13, your perception and thus your answers will be quite different than if you are 45, or even 65. Bear with me for some examples that will show exactly what I mean.

8

I remember, with a smile, a cartoon that I saw a long time ago in a medical journal. An ancient man, sitting on a bench and being questioned about his age, retorts with, "Which age do you mean? Anatomic, psychologic, physiologic, moral, or chronologic?"

My late mother-in-law, at the age of 81, met an old friend who was just turning 92. In describing the meeting, my mother-in-law took umbrage at the fact that I considered the two women contemporaries. "How can you compare *me* with *her*?" she asked haughtily. "*She's* middle-aged!"

The Bureau of Labor Statistics considers the category of "older worker" as anyone over 45!

Bernard Baruch once observed, "Old age is always 15 years older than I am."

Back in the mid '30s my mother was a radio soap opera addict. The daily fare included a continuing saga about a woman named Helen Trent. Each day, to the accompaniment of sobbing organ music, the announcer intoned, "Helen Trent . . . can a woman over 35 find romance?" It was some years later that I laughed out loud when I heard someone refer to *Helen Trent* as the program that gave virtue a bad name!

Enough? You have not even heard the beginning! I visited Florida several times in researching the retirement section of the book, and on one trip, while driving to a retirement condominium, I turned on the radio and heard a terse, important announcement:

> *. . . middle-aged hijacker of a Continental Airlines jet. Ninety passengers escaped through the rear exit. He is still holding seven passengers in first class and FBI agents are talking to the man, who is described as white, middle-aged, between the ages of 40 and 45 . . .*

My immediate reaction was that the announcer must be ten years old! There is always the reference to chronological age. The generation that proclaimed, "Never trust anyone over 30!" is now old enough to look around and shout, still more loudly, "Life begins at 40!" Sometimes it is countered by an older person's common sense, as when Gloria Swanson was quoted as saying, "I don't feel like 81—because I don't know how 81 feels!" How old, then, is old? What is middle age?

In fact, the theory of *life stages* is going the way of the Edsel, the Victrola, and the ice box. We make up a small, but vocal and perceptive, group that is beginning to realize that it is not only unfair, but also inaccurate, to categorize us in chronological stages, whether they are called passages, seasons, or transitional periods in our lives. It will make the writing of "life-style" books more difficult if we remove the boundaries, but remove them we must. The time is different. Things are not the same. And they will never go back to what they were.

Dr. Neugarten has given our historic time a most descriptive name in stating that this is an era of "age-irrelevance." And so it is. First of all, what we are at a specific age is very much dependent upon the society in which we live. It is just as important to think about the era in which we were born. Because the life span in colonial times was moderately short, our own early American society spawned politicians and diplomats who would have been in college or in graduate school were they living in our times. After all, if your projected life span were about 40, you had darned well better make your mark by the time you were 20! Had Mozart begun his career at 30, we would have had little of his music to listen to today.

So, in the first place, through medical advances, the years of potential have been increased. A good example is the minimal death rate of women in childbirth today as compared to what our grand-mothers had to contend with. The structured life style of not too many years ago—school, marriage, children, early aging, and death—has been drawn out to include decades of activity after the children are gone from the family home, resulting in much younger grandparents in many instances. They bring a freedom that comes with a society that has become more affluent than any that have preceded us. This allows us a flexibility of life style as never before. As Dr. Neugarten says, no one ever admonishes, "Act your age!" any longer.

In my research I found students at leading universities who were past the age of 80, some of them even trying for belated degrees. The mayor of a small Wisconsin city is at this writing barely 29 years old. Each year over 20,000 men over the age of 50 choose to become fathers, many of them for the first time. How nice for the world to discover that our generation is still sexual and lusty! Although Carl Jung was one of the first analytic thinkers to suggest that midlife was the time for max-imum potential and personality growth, our generation has borne out his optimism by the greatest surge of career changes and life-style metamorphoses in history. I am not quite sure, however, just what age Jung considered "midlife." Probably somewhere around 30!

Dr. Neugarten has also commented on the fact that a person need not be young because of age, nor does the word "old" connote a specific number of years. There are, she says, the "young old" as well as the "old old" and it all depends upon your state of mind. Think about your friends, as I did when I dedicated this book. None of those listed could, by any stretch of the imagination, be considered "old old," even though not one of them is below the age of 50 and most are well into their 60s.

But our society has been conditioned and it is not the first time. The Harris survey showed that 5 percent of the American public considers that a person reaches old age before turning 50! Another 16 percent felt that old age starts before 60. Soon we ourselves begin to believe all this, and we begin to act "old" before our time. If everyone says so, surely it must be true. They and we have been conditioned to think of physical changes as being the prime causes of our getting old— gray hair, wrinkles, brown spots on the skin.

We soon become the victims of the stereotypes imposed on us. It is how we *look* that makes us old, they say. And as we age, they treat us differently and think differently about us. And *we* believe it!

I go in to buy a roll of sewing thread, and the man bends to reach beneath the counter of his little shop. Possibly he is all of 45, and I hear him moan, "My back is killing me. I must be getting old!"

I walk uptown and meet an old friend by accident. I have not seen him in 20 years and, frankly, he has not aged badly at all, if I look at the physical signs. (Note that I, too, have commented upon the physical. Like you, I am a victim of ageism!) My friend is 64 and he says to me as he pulls off my winter hat and looks at my hair, "My, you've gotten gray!" (Did he expect that I had gotten gold?) "Well," he sighs sadly, "I guess we're all gettin' old."

I suppose we are, and right now I don't know of any solution to the aging process. But I am warmly reminded of the great Harry Hirschfield's statement at a testimonial dinner marking his 80th birthday: "How does it feel to be 80? Great, when you consider the alternative!"

# Nonsense, Claptrap, Stereotypes, and Moth-Eaten Myths

> *It is not aging that is at fault, but rather our attitude towards it.*
>
> *Cicero:*
> Treatise on Aging

**M**y dear friend Alex is now in his 70s—an active traveler, off-Broadway producer, art collector, and real estate executive. He tells about meeting a man on a crowded street in New York. Suddenly, out of the throng, the face appeared and Alex couldn't quite place where they had met before, nor just who the man was. It has happened to all of us—out of context, even a familiar face seems unplaceable. The two men greeted each other and Alex commented, still at a loss, "You know, there are *three* things that happen when you get older. The first thing is that you forget people's names. And—I can't remember the other two!"

I have used the story time and again when I have run into people by accident, and it is a superb icebreaker. But, if we analyze it, we realize that we are placing an unfair burden on the process of aging. We do it again, and yet again. We are getting older. It is accepted that we must, therefore, begin to forget things. It is the beginning of our own acceptance of "ageism" and it is just as insidious as the processes of racism and sexism. For *we* are the victims.

I am again guilty along with everyone else. I misplace my glasses (a reading crutch that I need more often now that my eyes are—naturally—aging). I blame it on creeping senility. The other night I took a wine glass and placed it somewhere in the house while I idly made notes for this morning's chapter of this book. Some spirit or hobgoblin stole it, though I discovered it several hours later where I had put it in the first place—right alongside my typewriter. I must, obviously, be in my "twilight years"!

The fact is that, if you were to observe the exact same things among your young friends or your children or grandchildren, you would probably pass these incidents off with a flippant comment that they have "too much on their minds" or they're "too busy" to think clearly. It is exactly this kind of destructive analysis that has plagued women and ethnic minorities in our society. In the corporate world, if a man is a driving, ambitious, single-minded workaholic who is demanding and rigid toward his subordinates, he is destined to become an executive vice-president as a reward for his personality and his efforts. Should a woman exhibit exactly the same type of personality, she will become known around the office as "an overbearing, arrogant bitch"!

It is easier to stereotype than to allow for differences. It is easier to do a survey about adolescents who are confined to an institution or older people in nursing homes than it is to probe the diversity that exists throughout our society. Unfortunately, as the myths are published, as the stereotypes are perpetuated by our employers, fellow employees, the general public, the media, and the folklore of aging, a most insidious thing happens to us. *We begin to believe them ourselves!* And, in the process, the myth becomes self-fulfilling and we, the victims, then help to sustain both the distorted facts and the nonsense. Well, just what are some of those myths? They begin to crop up as we enter middle age and, as we pass the point of no return at 65, they increase in quantity (if not in quality). They become even more destructive. Until now we have been normal, functioning, vital human beings. Age has come upon us. What are we like now?

Well, we are rigid and we reject innovation. Only the young (as everyone knows) are flexible and unflappable. We are impatient and cantankerous, of course, and we are moving rather quickly into our "second childhood."

We are all frail and in poor health or, at best, our health is failing rapidly. Certainly, we are absentminded and slow-witted. Worse, we are a burden to society, to our friends, and to our families. Worst of all, perhaps, is the fact that we are almost totally unproductive in our personal lives and in the business world. Make way for the young mind, and especially the young body!

And—ah yes—we are totally unsexual and dispassionate. And middle age is the time when most marriages break up in any case. The end result of all this is that we withdraw, to fade away and quietly disappear from living, unsung and barely remembered. And all this degeneration begins somewhere around the age of 40!

The theory of the "big lie" is no revelation to those who have lived as long as we have, especially through the propaganda of so many wars. Say a thing often enough and everyone will believe it. Say it loudly enough and it will drown out the feeble voice of truth. Soon the scapegoat joins the chorus and the fantasy becomes the inevitable reality.

One of the questions asked in the Harris study related to just how the public thought older people (over 65) spend *most* of their time. Look at the figures carefully, for some of the estimates were far off the reality.

> *Watching television:* Sixty-seven percent thought that we spend most of our time at the tube. Actually, 36 percent do that after the age of 65!
> *Sitting and thinking:* Sixty-two percent were convinced that we are posed as a series of Rodin statues, just a-settin' and a-thinkin'. The actual figure is 31 percent.
> *Taking a lot of walks:* Only 34 percent thought this, while 25 percent of us actually do spend our time on frequent walks.
> *Sleeping:* Here it was almost 40 percent versus 16 percent in actuality.

The most interesting answer came from 35 percent of those surveyed who thought that older people spend most of their time "just doing nothing." I would love to survey some of the young people to whom I've lectured at colleges across the country to find out just how many of them spend a good part of *their* time "doing nothing." Actually only 15 percent of people over 65 claim that "doing nothing" is the main pursuit of the day. That gives us 85 percent who must be doing something! And between ages 45 and 65, *almost all* of us are too busy to do nothing.

I am not the first author or researcher or sociologist to shout, "Bah! Humbug!" to all the nonsense that passes as gospel while masking the myths. The entire Harris study—all 245 pages of it—is devoted to an analysis of aging stereotypes such as image, the media, employment, finances, and expectation versus reality. In their own words, the researchers come to the conclusion that: "The picture drawn in the public's mind of old age and its problems is a gross distortion of what older people say they experience personally."

Most of the popular books I've read on the subject of middle age and old age, however, are frankly rather depressing. While starting out to disprove the stereotypes, they end up by going along with many of them, from "midlife crisis" to menopausal depression, leading eventually to disintegration and suicidal tendencies.

One of the most upbeat books on the subject, however, is Alex Comfort's *A Good Age* (Crown, New York, 1976), in which he calls the process I've been describing as "sociogenic aging." It is the role which society imposes upon people as they reach a specific chronological age, in spite of all the current talk of age-irrelevance and our own feelings about having reached middle age. If you are 65 you must, of course, retire. If you are 45 you have reached well into midlife, and you must be unemployable or forgetful or unsexual.

Nina Kenny of the Colonial Penn Group (which insures only older Americans) told me about a newspaper story when I interviewed her for the information in this chapter about older drivers. A gentleman was crossing Market Street in Philadelphia. He had just turned 65 and was on his way to a birthday luncheon with his son. Suddenly he felt his son's hand as it took his elbow in a firm grip and guided him across the street. He turned and asked, "What are you doing?" The son's rejoinder was, "Well, you're 65, and I'm helping you across the street." To which the father, somewhat annoyed, retorted, "You didn't help me across the street when I was 64. Why are you helping me at 65?"

It is out of this sea of myths and stereotypes that the problems of aging emerge. And though we may be 45 or 50 or not yet at our 65th birthday, it begins to affect us at an early stage. Just look, if you will, at the advertising and note the number of times that the copy mentions "young." It is no wonder that many of our feelings about ourselves begin to reflect society's absurdities, even while we are just entering the road of middle age. If by chance we should disagree with what is being said and written in the media, we generally pass it off and say, "Well, I'm an *exception!*"

A young acquaintance of mine was holding forth one evening as only the young can do—secure, rigid, and totally incorrect. (Note, if you will, my stereotype of the young. Is this known as "youthism"?) She claimed that every bad driver she had ever seen was an older person. They held up traffic, did dangerous things, and generally made her life miserable on the highway. I pointed out to her that I thought the accident rate of younger drivers was higher than that of the older driver. Of course, she asked for proof.

Soon after that I took the train to Philadelphia to speak with Nina Kenny of Colonial Penn, since insurance companies are not about to take chances on bad risks. There are more than 40 million licensed drivers over the age of 50, and 10 million are over the age of 65, she told me. In all, they represent 30 percent of all drivers in the country. In spite of what my young friend says, this older driving group is involved in less than 20 percent of the accidents. The under-30 age group—my young acquaintance's contemporaries—*is responsible for twice as many accidents.*

Most of us older drivers are well aware of our limitations, such as diminished eyesight, or perhaps a small loss of hearing, and, as a result, we compensate for them. Many of us avoid driving at dawn and dusk and, after retirement, the need to drive distances seems to diminish in any case.

I never did bring up the subject again, but the final curtain was lowered about a month later in Portland, Oregon, when I heard an early-morning call-in show while I was dressing for an appointment. The young MC (who also must have been ten years old) asked the question, "Well, what about all those old geezers on the highway?" An Oregon state trooper called in to answer, "Older people are rarely convicted of speeding, and rarely obliged to take driver training programs." He did suggest, however, that eye exams be made mandatory.

So much for another myth. And as each of the stereotypes is examined, it evaporates like dew in the sun. There is the myth that middle age is the time when most marriages break up. Before I go any further, did you nod in agreement? Well, it just is not true. The divorce rate is actually highest in teen-age marriages, and it gradually decreases and goes steadily downhill through the years.

The middle-aged person who is productive, sexual, affluent, independent, and very strong is not the exception. If I have come to one firm, irrevocable conclusion on this journey, it is that we are *all* exceptions. As mature people, we are a more heterogeneous group than any other in this country. Indeed, it is the *young* who are probably most apt to adopt the habits and protective colorations of conformity. Do you remember the "uniform" when you were in high school? In my generation it was saddle shoes and team sweaters.

It was the young people of the '60s who became the hippies and the flower children because of the sameness of their dress, their language, and their philosophies (not to mention their almost universal white, middle-class backgrounds). In the arena of revolution for the young, there is security in sameness.

It is only as we progress from youth to maturity that we begin to be different, individual. How ironic, then, that so much of the country's stereotypical thinking should be directed toward the middle-aged, the aged, and the very process of aging.

The generalizations about aging present a totally negative view of our lives, just as many of the myths portray middle age as a time when we are all put out to pasture, to gambol on the lawn of the retirement village of our choice. Each as a totality is incorrect, and both are harmful to a fuller understanding of the process and the changes in aging. The list could continue on and on: Older people are all senile. Middle-aged people all become politically conservative. Older people really don't want to be with the young but like to live among themselves. And, of course—"you can't teach an old dog new tricks!"

But is it changing? That is, after all, what this book is about. Everything in life changes, though not always for the best. Slowly the myths and the misconceptions are giving way to a more realistic outlook that views aging as a normal event in the life cycle. More important, perhaps, is the beginning of an awareness that the aging population of this country is a significant and valuable natural resource. We are beginning to discover, also, that we do not age in a vacuum, but that *all* our experiences in life, including our attitudes while still very young, will determine whether we get to the age of 50 or 60 as one of the "young old" or the "old old." Above all, if we have reached this mountaintop in our lives, we are certainly pretty good survivors!

# Is Gerontophobia
# a Curable Disease?

*Despise not thy mother when she is old.*
                                    Proverbs 23:22

For a very short time I seriously considered omitting any interview with Maggie Kuhn for this book. I had heard so much about her, collected many of her articles and statements in my research files, watched her on television, read about her in the newspapers and newsmagazines, and even discovered that she had written an introduction to a book dedicated to the good health of older Americans. Falling victim to an author's perversity, I was on the verge of deciding that Maggie and her organization, the Gray Panthers, had been "overdone" and anything that I might add would be extraneous and repetitive. Such a decision would have been a sad mistake and I would have lost both a remarkable interview and an extraordinary personal experience.

"Gerontophobia has reached epidemic proportions. It's a massive social disease!" She said it with conviction, as she says everything that involves her, and that encompasses the process of aging and the distortion of that process in the minds of our society. She went on: "In

18

children, it's a fear of old people—and there's a good deal of evidence that children's books and stories for little ones begin to infect them with a fear of old people. Old people are presented as witches—troublesome, unpleasant characters. And the little girl on TV says, 'Why grandma, what are those brown spots on your hands? They're ugly!' and grandma says, 'Yes, they're ugly, but I'm rubbing them with Porcelana.' Now, there's a little kid who obviously loves her grandma, who is reinforcing the self-contempt that grandma feels. I hate those hands! I hate me! It may be a trivial aspect, but that's self-rejection. It's very deep. And our children reinforce it because they themselves are infected with gerontophobia."

We sat in the living room of the old, rambling, creaky house that had seen better days. It was raining in Philadelphia and I was glad I had made the trip. We laughed each time the electricity in the building went off and then back on again a few moments later. And we sat on wooden, hand-carved, straight-backed chairs for almost two hours and we talked and we laughed—and became angry together.

"Think of what gerontophobia does to children and young people," she continued. "Young people infected with it have no future. And middle-aged people are very afraid, if they admit it. It's a Western disease. It's a disease of the advanced countries. We've all got it. The super-technologically advanced countries, including Japan. We've substituted material values. We've made a God of technology." She sat back.

How does one describe Maggie Kuhn as she does battle well into her 75th year? She is small and slender, with gray hair and a tiny frame, but with a remarkably commanding presence, as anyone who has seen her speak will attest. I had expected her to arrive at that old house that was Gray Panther headquarters and come bursting through the door, a firebrand who would rattle the windows and shake the chandeliers. But she walked up the wet path gently, carrying an umbrella, preceded by her young assistant, Cindy Traub, and there was the feeling that I had known her for a very long time. She is poised, beautiful, articulate, intense, and caring—and very impatient with things that don't get done, impatient with people, especially people of *our* age, who don't do anything about improving their situation. She dismisses middle-aged and older people who cry about their plight as "wrinkled babies." She joins those who really care enough to do something, along with the young, to fight as Youth and Age in Action. I shall speak more of the Gray Panthers in Chapter 20, but I came away with a strong sense of "self," and I sent my check for membership in the Gray Panthers about two weeks later.

Possibly it would matter less if you and I were part of a declining segment, a generation that represented only a small percentage of the American population. But if ever there was a group to whom the census statistics are vital, it is our invisible generation. Older Americans—and that includes us, like it or not—are the fastest growing minority group in the country. The cult of youth may well be on its way out. Within just a few years you and I will be over 65—some of us more quickly than others, of course—but instead of being part of a diminishing minority, we will eventually outnumber the young!

By the year 2000 the generation that said, "You can't trust anyone over 30," will be in their 50s!

Back in 1900 only 1 person out of 25 was over the age of 65. The ratio today is 1 in 9. By the year 2000, when we will all be there, the ratio will rise to 1 out of 8!

If we project all this to the year 2030, the ratio jumps to 1 of every 6 Americans over the age of 65, and if we add the people of the 40-to-65 age group, the total comes to slightly under 50 million people.

All this translates to the fact that the median age of our country keeps going up. The first census was taken in America in 1790 and, at that time, about 50 percent of all our citizens were under 16 years of age. By 1970 the median age had risen to 28 and it is slightly more than 30 at the time of this writing. But by the year 2030 it will be 40. The toddlers of the post-World War II "baby boom" will have turned gray, and we will see a vast increase in both the numbers and the proportion of middle-aged and older people, in relation to the total American population.

The increase in our numbers is beginning to have a serious effect on our social programs, our economic lives, and our personal view of ourselves; it has already altered our family relationships and our career roles as well as career goals. Finally, and most important, if the portrayals of middle age and the process of aging continue to be exaggerated and distorted negatively, they cannot help but have a deleterious effect upon our young people as well as upon ourselves, in that they may well instill in our sons and daughters a deep-seated fear of growing older.

I said early on that I am not a Pollyanna. At least I try not to be. We—all of us—do think about aging. We would be fools if the subject totally slipped our minds. There are reminders every day of our lives and most of them are amusing incidents, though admittedly we react to them with a start. The view from here is that we think more about the years that are left to us than about how long ago we were born. The police officer on our beat begins to look very young. My cameraman turns to me as I describe an old film just rerun on television and he asks, "Zasu Pitts? Who's Zasu Pitts?" It bothers me enough so that I call him late one night and tell him to tune in to channel 4 so that he can see "who's Zasu Pitts"! An entire generation has barely, if ever, heard of Shirley Temple or Chester Morris, or even less likely, of my childhood love, Helen Twelvetrees. Of course, it happens to all of us.

In the writing of a book the period of pregnancy, followed by terrible labor pains, and the eventual "unnatural birth" of words on paper can make an author a difficult person to be with. Not only have I researched this book quite formally over this past year, but I find that I constantly question my friends in every social situation. Just a few hours ago, while still in the throes of this chapter, I stopped by to speak to my friend Ernie, who lives near the ocean, and to share a glass of wine with him and another fishing companion, George. Both are "middle-aged" by any standards, which means that they are somewhere over 35, but closer to 55 or 60. We spoke of that first time, that first revelation, when suddenly we realized that we were getting older. It is as vivid in everyone's memory as the loss of virginity.

"I think," Ernie recounted, "that it happened twice in the same week. The first time was when someone at work called me 'Sir.' " The second event happened some years back when his teen-age children were having a rather noisy party. Ernie, just 40, became annoyed at the shouting and the screaming and the raucous music and he came downstairs to demand that they quiet down. One young man turned and ran across the lawn, brandishing a bottle of beer and uttering loud Indian war whoops. Ernie gave chase and caught him in ten quick steps. The young man, obviously under the influence of alcohol, laughed uproariously and yelled to his friends, "Watch out for the *old guy!* He can run like a jackrabbit!"

We all laughed as I recounted how Gail Sheehy had written that middle age begins in the 30s, bringing forth an expletive from one of the women in the group, whose age is about 50 and who still feels that she has ten years to go before entering midlife. George thought a while, sipping his wine, and then quietly told us that he never really thinks about aging except when he realizes that the partners in his law firm, who hired him 29 years ago, were the same age then as he is now—and he thought of *them* as old men the day of his interview!

I feel that all this is perfectly normal, perfectly natural, a healthy awareness of the change that is taking place all through our lives, especially as we grow and mature. We have lived through more and have more experience, as well as an innate ability to evaluate what we have gone through and what is yet to come. The examples that most of us give are merely recognition that there *is* a gap between generations. It exists on a cultural level and on a social plane and, certainly, the emotional distance is enormous. I am not certain that there is a distance on a financial level, because it is my observation that our younger people are, in general, quite affluent. Somehow they don't seem to have the underlying feeling of financial insecurity that most of our Depression-generation peers carry with them. But on all other levels we may as well face it—we *are* different. It would help some, however, if both age groups tried to understand each other. And herein lies the problem of creeping gerontophobia.

The examples that my friends gave are quite harmless to them, a nod to the inevitability of aging. They are, as I said, merely musings and an awareness of change. But the insidious and destructive societal pressures in relation to middle-age and aging are quite another story. The moment we are affected by the pressures from the outside and begin to doubt ourselves, the "problems" of aging begin. Take, for example, the subject of gray hair.

One of the people I interviewed for this book told me that she had discovered her first gray hairs the day she was 23 and suddenly, that morning, when she looked in her mirror, the world began to change for her. She was becoming middle-aged! How many friends have you known who felt the same thing? Possibly it even happened to you at a tender age. It is not to be passed off lightly, because you (and I?) have just contracted the first symptoms of the dread disease, gerontophobia. Why, after all, is gray hair so damned awful? It doesn't change your heartbeat. It shouldn't change your sex life—in fact, it may even proclaim you as a more experienced partner.

The answer is obvious, and part of it was angrily commented upon at a recent White House Conference on Older Women held in Des Moines. One of the workshops was called, "Images of Growing Older Female," and the discussion centered upon the differences in how a man and a woman are perceived by society after the gray has begun to take over. One of the comments was that "a man with gray hair is perceived to be sexy, having money and power." To which another woman added, "But a woman with gray hair is perceived as sitting by the fireplace rocking, with a white cap on her head."

If all were well, if gerontophobia were not a social disease, the discovery of a few strands of gray hair would be accepted, as would letting the entire head of hair go gray and natural. And that would be that. But the pressures of society, our families, the media, and ourselves demand that we do something about it. Clairol insists that we have a "coloring experience." The family, the children, insist that we look too old, asking us when we plan to "do something about it." The slogan, "Does she or doesn't she?" is obviously being answered rather resoundingly with, "She damned well doesn't!" But the arm-twisting continues unabated. I read recently that Barbara Bush, the wife of the Vice-President, receives letters from strangers asking her why she doesn't consider a "younger" color. (Green, perhaps? Or purple?)

The revolt against all this is happening very slowly. Some women are rebelling and letting it "all hang out." In the business world, especially, women who seem to feel more secure and are on the executive level are refusing to color their hair. My wife, Sheryl, saw the first flecks of gray when she was 17 and she never did anything about it, becoming a beautiful, totally gray-haired woman at the age of 35. The ironic thing about all this is that people come up to Sheryl on the street or on the bus to ask, "Who colors your hair?" Sarcastically, but with a smile, she answers, "Haven't you heard—it's that new Clairol color, *Going Gray!*"

For the rest of us there are still the problems of job hunting in later life and competing with the young, who have not yet discovered the first tell-tale flecks when they look in their mirrors in the morning. For out there in the real world the fears of aging still exist.

Certainly it is time that we begin thinking less about what we have lost and what we are losing by entering middle age, and more about who we are and what we are gaining in new freedoms during these years. Attitudes must change, and in the next chapter I will discuss just how we begin to change them and just who (and what) our targets are. There is no doubt that gerontophobia lives. But, given the proper treatment, it is not fatal and, indeed, it can be cured!

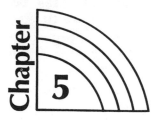

# The Middle-Age "Hit List"

> *Life'd not be worth livin' if we didn't keep our inimies.*
>
> Finley Peter Dunne:
> Mr. Dooley in Peace & War

"We're stuck with a situation of self-fulfilling prophecies . . . granted that we are our own worst enemies, our next worst enemies are our families—and our physicians! Certainly, that's plenty of enemies to have!"

I laughed. The telephone conversation to Portland, Maine, had gone on for well over half an hour at that point and it was destined for still another 30 minutes. The vitality emanating over the line was the best thing that had happened to me that day. Though my original reason for telephoning Marty Knowlton was to learn more about how he founded Elderhostel (Chapter 18), he and I were soon caught up in the conversation of middle-aged peers probing deeply to find out just who they are; covering the common ground of experience, laughing at ourselves and at the society in which we live, discussing our future plans in teaching, writing, traveling. Most of all, I was charmed by the idea of his list of "enemies." It made me feel almost a part of a previous presidential administration that was supposed to have kept its secret "hit list." The only difference was, I suppose, that the President's men had not put *themselves* at the top of *their* list.

Ever since Dr. Robert N. Butler of the National Institute on Aging coined the word "ageism," it has become more and more evident that many of the middle-aged and elderly are *themselves* as prejudiced as any younger group of people. It stands to reason, does it not, that if we have learned all our lives to have a negative attitude toward aging, we will carry that same attitude into our later years. When I spoke to Marty I had already discovered for myself just how deep-seated this self-hate had become in our society, in spite of the fact that my own friends exhibited none of it and that they were the most active, vital people I had ever known. And yet all were middle-aged and growing older along with the rest of society. But the *family*? The family as an enemy? The sacrosanct, American, true-red-white-and-blue family?

Marty roared. "*Families*? Well, God, how old are you?"

"Fifty-seven," I answered.

"Well, you're old enough! I'm 60. Suppose you or I, in the event that we were free—that we had no wife, were widowed or divorced— suppose we started to go out and began dating a woman. Suppose we decided to stay away for the weekend!"

I contemplated the situation and muttered some innocuous re- mark while Marty continued and the telephone shook: "*Why, our fam- ilies would be outraged!*"

I nodded and he went on, warming up as the Bell Telephone clock ticked away. "Oh God, the kids really set a terrible standard of conformity. I use that because it's a rather striking example. You may have a daughter or a son who's living with someone, living without bothering to get married, and *you* decide to go off for a weekend with a person of *your* age. Good God! Children in particular seem to get quite outraged at parents who fail to conform. Now, mind you, they don't *want* you to be sick, they don't *want* you to show signs of mental aberration, but they behave as though that's exactly how they *do* think of you!"

By the time Marty had finished that portion of his tirade, I began to resent the children we'd never had. How dare they think that way? He was right; he was very right! Having taken care of our kids quite properly, we proceeded to the next enemy on the list, *our physicians*.

This is a terribly difficult and complex area for someone of my background to treat. Like you, I was brought up in the era of house calls and the adulation of the family physician as a minor (or major) god. When my dear mother spoke of "the Specialist," there was a feeling that we were to face to the East and genuflect. The subject is so complex, in fact, that I shall devote the greater part of a later chapter to problems of health, the doctor, and the responsibility that we all have for our own health. But, still retaining a part of my heritage of guilt, I envision a fantasy in which my family doctor (whom I love) is saying to me, "If *I* am your enemy, as you proclaimed in your book, then *you* are mine—and I will not treat you for the terminal disease with which you are afflicted!" In spite of this, I grit my teeth and push onward.

From a very pragmatic view, however, I wonder why we expect our physicians to feel any different from the other elements of our society. If ageism affects even the aging, why should it not affect the doctors? They live with us too. Why should we expect more from them than we do from ourselves? Perhaps because we cannot bear to shatter the idols to whom we look when we need help.

"Yes, but if you could just get doctors to say that this is a disease, but it just happens to be with an older person," Marty went on, warming to this new subject, "if you could do that, you'd have taken a mile-long stride. But in fact what the doctor says is, 'This is an older person and there's not much we can do for an older person anyway.' You still have a formidable number of physicians who frequently use the diagnosis of 'senescence.'"

I was reminded of the story told again and again, in various forms, of the old gentleman who visited his doctor complaining of a deep pain in his shoulder. "What can you expect," the doctor says, "You're 97 years old." The elderly gentleman retorts, rather haughtily, "My *other* shoulder is 97 years old too, and *it* doesn't hurt!" I found the story again in Alex Comfort's *A Good Age* (with a 104-year-old knee) and it was told to me two weeks later by my friend Rudy (with a 95-year-old foot). You can pass it on with whatever part of the anatomy you wish; it makes an excellent point.

No doubt about it, the aging population feels that it is being "ripped off" by the medical profession. Marty Knowlton suggested that, when I visit the Elderhostels the next summer, I speak with the elderly students at the noon meal. He guaranteed that the subject of health and medicine would come up, "and you will hear expressed what can only be described as a *hatred* for doctors, a terribly bitter hatred. 'Nobody cares about the aging; the doctors don't like them.' And I think our grounds for a dislike of the medical profession are very well perceived, indeed." (I did visit and they did bear him out.)

We ended our phone conversation some 30 minutes later, promising to contact each other if our busy schedules permitted. My note pad would be deciphered later in the quiet of my office, alone with my typewriter—my illegible scrawl was eventually decoded to read, "Three enemies: self, family, physician." There simply had to be more, even though Marty felt that three were quite enough.

In the months that followed I began to suspect that my "hit list" was incomplete. Somehow, I felt sure that there must be other "enemies" of the aging. I mulled over the three on the list, "self, family, physician," then I penciled in one more: *the corporation.*"

The list was filling out and I felt like Edward G. Robinson as "Little Caesar," deciding who was next. (Thank goodness we are all old enough to remember Edward G. Robinson!)

It is not only that the American corporation is youth-oriented. The hidden slogans, "Make way for the young ones coming up and give them a chance" and "Step aside, retire, you've played your role," are actually very practical prejudices. The corporation can ostensibly justify catering to the young while rejecting or casting aside the older worker. It has nothing to do with an older worker's lack of efficiency, as we shall see later on. It is another of the pragmatic realities brought forth by the accountants and the comptrollers. It's more economical! It costs less!

Primarily, the young worker or the employee just starting out receives less pay than someone with seniority. The additional expenses borne by the corporation on account of its staff are minimal when someone is under 25, rather than over 50. Health insurance, pension funds, and disability insurance costs are all lower for the young employee than for the older one.

It was recently borne out for me again. My small corporation had grown large enough for me to hire a full-time, permanent employee. I filled out the necessary papers, filed the forms with the federal government and the state, and discussed the plan with my insurance agent, my pension advisor, and my accountant. The fact that this young woman is eminently qualified for the job, has just the right amount of experience (much of it with me in the past), speaks five languages, and can handle a film crew anywhere in the world seemed to make no difference. The key question seemed to be, "How old is she?" And the reaction to my answer was, "Great! She's young enough to make the additional expenses minimal."

Multiply this, if you will, by the 10,000 or perhaps 50,000 people in a large company. The total can be substantial. The result is the same—the old must make way for the young. For example, a new pension plan is not vested until four or five years after a worker begins the job. It is possible that the entire sum will be returned to the corporation if the worker leaves before that time. In dealing with the 50-year-old, early retirement is a good way for the corporation to cut back on pension expenditures.

There is another way in which some corporations play the villain, and I think it is tightly tied to the problems of ageism in the company. In all the years of dealing with America's top companies and in reading the business sections of newspapers and magazines, I have seldom seen an acceptance of responsibility for the human, physical problems created by a manufacturing process or a corporate philosophy. Blanket denial is the typical response to the accusation of being a bad corporate citizen.

Of course, not all corporations are guilty of this, and many for which I have produced films in these past 35 years are very much concerned with the environment, the inner city, and the rights of minorities. Their public image is also their private one, and for that they are to be congratulated.

But when we read of a defective product being recalled, it is generally at the urging of the government. I keep waiting for someone to take responsibility for the problems of lung cancer and heart disease that have been placed at the doorstep of the tobacco industry. I wonder when a concerned corporate citizen will step up and genuinely respond to the Love Canals, the PCB dumping, and the poisons that pollute the rivers and lakes. The answer that "at the time our company did it, it was the state of the art" somehow doesn't seem good enough. The cancer in the asbestos industry, the brown lung of the cotton mills, the black lung of the mines, the unsafe machines on the assembly lines are all a part of the picture. And the answer to all this is exactly the same as the answer to the ageism which characterizes American industry. It is more economical to deny that it exists. To admit blame is to be forced to pay. If these are our good corporate citizens, why should we expect them to treat the middle-aged worker any differently than they treat the environment? The appalling thing to me, in addition, is that these same executive denials are made by people just like *us*, who live in our communities, who have families just as vulnerable to the poisons in our atmosphere and our workplace, and who can "put on another hat" when they enter their offices. I have never been able to understand that.

If it will help at all, you can be sure of two things. First of all, it is much worse in many other countries. There are cities I have visited all over the world where the smog and the smoke and the carcinogens seem to enter your hotel room once you awaken in the morning and open the window to greet the hazy sun, fighting its way in through the gloom.

Second, you can be certain that it will get worse. The country is moving more and more toward a laissez-faire attitude in terms of our business community. Corporations, it has been decreed, will now begin policing themselves—no more government interference. We can forget the reasons for the policing in the first place, forget the way Pittsburgh looked before the new industrial laws were instituted, and we can bury Love Canal again. It will be like letting the Ku Klux Klan investigate a lynching in Alabama in 1933!

Once again I looked at my list: "self, family, physician, corporation." One more to go—another member of the "hit list" bent on making us invisible. But, just because it is last on the list, don't ever feel that it is, therefore, least. Let me introduce you to a not-very-good friend of ours: *the media.*

# The Medium Is the Mirror

> *Thou art unseen, but yet I hear thy shrill delight.*
> *Percy Bysshe Shelley:*
> The Cloud

I will admit right at the start that it is sometimes too easy to condemn the press, radio, movies, or television for our invisibility. For too many generations the media have been condemned for all manner of social, economic, and sexual ills. In my mother's time, her mother condemned the "dime novel" for instilling hopeless romantic dreams in a young girl's head. The era of yellow journalism, still with us today in many of our newspapers and magazines, has been cited as spreading crime and violence through the reportage and glorification of the convulsions that wrack a changing society.

More recently our library books have again become the targets of the wrath of parents who hold the publishing industry responsible for the absence of worthwhile values in their children, for sexual promiscuity, smoking marijuana, abortion, rape, and lack of ambition. I read with horror recently of a Midwest group which was taking books off the shelves of the local libraries because the books were spreading the heresy of "humanism" (whatever is meant by that) as well as birth control and other distortions too numerous to mention. One of the books I grew up with, *Catcher in the Rye,* is no longer there. (And thousands of kids are missing the wonderful Holden Caulfield.) *Brave New World* has been banished. You may be certain that, if society is sick, the media will be blamed for spreading the plague, whether it be through television, advertising, newspapers, motion pictures, or the books we read.

The fact is that much of what we *choose* to read is rubbish and most of what we watch on television is neutral. Every sizable city in the country boasts a daily newspaper whose best attribute is that it is just thick enough and wide enough to wrap the morning trash for collection. But I tread very lightly in one important area when I speak of the media as an enemy of the aging.

I do not believe in censorship. I do not believe that we should muzzle any part of the media. I am fully aware that the rights of the parents of whom I speak are as sacrosanct as my own—*but only in making themselves heard and felt,* and not in any way impinging upon my choice of what I read or what I view or how I think. "Your freedom ends where my nose begins," Voltaire said. And I mutter a loud "amen"!

The media, with all the warts and flaws of any institution run by human beings, may be no more guilty of perpetuating the myths and stereotypes of aging than other segments of our society. Indeed, is it fair to blame all our problems on just one element that mirrors what all of us seem to think about ourselves?

One of the most interesting conclusions of the Harris study was that, generally speaking, the public is *not* critical of the way the media portray the people of our generations. The media themselves point to this conclusion when faced with complaints. They tell us that they merely reflect the stereotypes and myths that are *already* a part of the public image. Certainly a possibility. But does that relieve the media of all responsibility for the prevailing impression? Am I being unfair when I declare the media responsible in large part for distorting our image? Am I unfair when I designate them as an integral part of my "hit list"? Not by a long shot!

This is a society based upon a strong media presence. A majority of our citizens cannot remember the era before television. Because of our high literacy rate, newspapers, magazines, and books play an important role in the dissemination not only of facts, but of pseudo-facts and myths as well. An institution as pervasive and as powerful as the American media cannot be allowed to excuse itself with, "We're only a mirror. We give the public what it wants."

Ironically, the middle-aged—our generation—run the media. (And they are, by happenstance, mostly men.) Though I was raised in a much more naive era, when we expected some good to come from the people in power, I see that it is only pressure brought by large segments of the marketplace that gets their attention. It is no different in the political arena. We naively expect an aged President to have some compassion for an aging population. Instead, we find that when Social Security is endangered, he seems indifferent. Our basic source of income in our later years can be saved only through the hue and cry of what the politicians derogatorily call "special interest groups"—namely, *us*.

# Television: The Distorted Image

My television set is still an old, decrepit black-and-white model dating from about 1954. I see no need to change it; it still works. I do not feel as my father did when he got his first color set. I entered the room to exclaim, "Dad, the baseball diamond is all blue!" Barely turning around to answer, he retorted, "So what! It's in *color*!" The only time I see color television is in hotel rooms in distant cities while dressing for the day. In those early morning hours, as I watch what passes for discussion by uninformed actors who have only the barest acquaintance with the material they are presenting, I vow again to retain my black-and-white set until it self-destructs. Besides, the old set is one of those models which can be operated by remote control and, late at night when I get very angry, I can simply shoot a beam at it and shut it off completely. What an unmatched sense of power!

I mention all this to put this chapter into its proper perspective. It is not, by any stretch of the imagination, an objective view of television. Neither is it an overall indictment of television. It is, rather, a selective compilation of the things that relate only to us—the middle-aged and aging in our population. I leave the overall analyses to those who spend more time than I do in front of the set.

Back in the late '40s, when I was a young television director, I gave a speech to a group of men at a local social club. In awesome tones I informed them that we had "over 100,000 television sets in the United States and the next year the number might very well double!" I smile now as I write this, for the statistics have long since arrived at amazing totals. According to A. C. Neilsen & Company, almost 78 *million* households now have TV sets, with an average of 1.75 sets per household. That does not include those in bars, lounges, airports, or hospitals, or portable sets. There are over 700 television stations now operating (and the number is growing rapidly with new cable channels opening every day), beaming nearly 5 *million hours* of television programming each year. And the bottom line is money.

In his marvelous little book, *Television and the Aging Audience* (University of Southern California Press, 1980), Dr. Richard H. Davis of the Ethel Percy Andrus Gerontology Center defines television as "pop art . . . aimed toward the masses. Further, it is mass-produced by profit-minded entrepreneurs solely for the gratification of a paying mass audience. . . . Television, which is supposed to be free and operating in the 'interest, convenience, and necessity of the people,' is actually the servant of the merchandisers."

Maybe we are a viable and growing market. Maybe we do represent the majority of prime-time viewers. But that is not the deciding factor. It is how the marketer thinks of his audience that eventually determines the programming, casting, image, or myth to be broadcast. Some time ago the brilliant *New York Times* columnist Russell Baker began his weekly satire with the statement that "the faces of television newswomen are never wrinkled." He went on to explain that he did not include the *men,* such as Walter Cronkite. Their faces, he wrote, "always seem to have arrived fresh from the presser two seconds ahead of the camera." Imagine your reactions if one evening, on prime-time network news, a woman in her 60s appeared, delivering the anchor spot commentary for one of the major stations in your city. No more Rather, Cronkite, Chancellor, Safer—but an attractive gray-haired, articulate, intelligent older woman! Possibly you would nod and say, "Why not?" But the perception of the network executive is different: "Who'd believe the news coming from a little old lady who could be your grandmother?"

In fact, not only is the suggestion fantasy, but exactly the opposite seems to be happening on television. The aging population, if you were to believe that flickering purveyor of misinformation, is a *vanishing* breed. Look only at the dramatic shows on television, those great "slice-of-life" hours that communicate the shallowness of our lives when the schedule is not busy with "T and A" ("tits and ass" in TV's charming executive vernacular—more modestly known as "jiggle shows"); only 3 percent of the major characters on the shows are old.

*📖*Old *women* account for less than 1 percent of the major characters on these shows.
*📖*Old *black women* are generally depicted only as victims or corpses.

I would be as breathless as a "Pepsi-generation" teen-ager if I had been the first to discover all this. There have been incredibly deep and reflective studies of the problems of television and its portrayal of the middle-aged and aging. Not only is the study by Dr. Davis a complete and well-structured report on the problem, but the Media Watch of the Gray Panthers, the White House Mini-Media Conference (January 1981), and Dr. George Gerbner, Dean of the University of Pennsylvania's Annenberg School of Communications (and his staff) have all issued complete and damning in-depth studies on the imbalance of ages on television, and the destructive role that stereotyping plays in programming.

Dr. Gerbner sampled 1,365 programs involving almost 17,000 characters, covering television plays, movies, cartoons, situation comedies, and crime-action shows. Immediately, he found that *more than half* of the TV population was between the ages of 25 and 45. The only statistic that makes me feel that we are not alone is that the under-18 group, who make up about 30 percent of our population, are represented by 8 percent of the fictional characters.

*📖*Between 40 and 65, the *men* more or less hold their own.
*📖*Aging men begin to represent power, political clout, and sophisticated, gray-haired affluence. Frequently in prime time the aging man is represented as a despicable villain, but be grateful for the little things—at least he *is* represented.

In direct contrast to what actually happens in our society, where the women begin to outnumber the men—television gives us the opposite picture.

*📖*The middle-aged woman begins to disappear from the screen as she turns the corner at 40 or 45.

Thus, if there is extreme justification in crying out against a state of invisibility, the woman of our generation must certainly have an inside track. She begins to disappear very much as though the antenna had been turned on the wrong axis and away from the beamed signal. And no amount of adjusting the dials will ever bring her back.

Dr. Davis explains it only too well. "Society's regard for an individual appears to be in direct ratio to his contribution to the gross national product. . . . Individual appeal (sometimes confused with worth) is measured on a value scale of attractiveness. The best women are beautiful and young. The best men are virile and young. . . . In TV, however, men become more powerful as they grow older. They control the money." And here, of course, television does mirror our society, does it not?

But it is not only the "disappearing act" that disturbs the researchers and the sociologists. Even worse than the disturbing statistics is *the way* in which television represents the aging portion of our population. The Annenberg report states, "More older characters are treated with disrespect than are characters in any other age group. About 70 percent of older men and more than 80 percent of older women are not held in high esteem or treated courteously, a very different pattern of treatment than that found for younger characters. . . . A much larger proportion of older characters than younger characters are portrayed as eccentric or foolish. A greater proportion of older women than older men—two-thirds compared to about half—are presented as lacking common sense, acting silly, or being eccentric. This male-female distinction is not salient in other age groups."

There is an interesting and ironic twist to the presentation of the aging man on television, however. It is true that the role of our male age group is frequently associated with power. But before you, sir, explode with pride, read on. The Annenberg report also concludes that "old men have the highest ratio of fatal victimization among all male age groups. Old men in television drama, especially when in a major, prime-time, serious role, are more likely to be evil than any other age group. Evil must have power to be credible. But in a world of happy endings, evil must also perish—hence the high ratio of old men who are killed."

There is an interesting exception to all this, though it does not take place during prime-time hours. On the daytime radio and television serials—the soap operas—younger characters are depicted more negatively than older characters. The latter are often the sympathetic friends, older business people, even older women. The younger ones seem to do nothing but get into some sort of trouble, depending upon what is currently "in" at that moment—abortion, pregnancy, rape, herpes, or stealing someone else's spouse.

If we turn to the area of television news and documentaries, the coverage is even more strongly unbalanced, since most of the reporting is concerned with the elderly *poor*. What follows from that is a picture that is even more distorted—the institutionalization of the elderly, the retired couples on welfare, the unemployed, and the destitute. Economic problems, poor health, loneliness. The decrepit, unloved, unwanted, hungry, suicidal. No matter what demographics exist to prove the contrary, this is our television picture of the aging.

It is no wonder that, according to both the Harris study and the Annenberg report, the more people watch television—and especially the younger generations—the more they tend to perceive old people in generally negative and unfavorable terms. "Those who watch more television believe that people (especially women) become old earlier in life," concludes the Harris study.

I think that one of the most astounding and revealing things is that the researchers did not find "watching television to be associated with *any* positive images of older people." One researcher claimed that the pattern was creating "symbolic annihilation" of our generations.

Is there hope? The damage has been done for so many years that even the public sees nothing wrong with the image being presented by television. And the networks, in turn, raise their halo-crowned, antenna-shaped heads and innocently say, "Why are you picking on *us*?"

For some years now the Public Broadcasting System has been producing a program called "Over Easy," devoted entirely to the issues, concerns, and challenges of the older American. It is at least an attempt at programming for our generation; but it is still a small dent in the system. Somehow I find myself comparing it to the years of pointing to Jackie Robinson and Ralph Bunche as examples of racial equality in America. There are dozens of children's shows on television—cartoons and Captain Kangaroos and the rest—yet we are expected to rejoice because we have *a* show of our own. And what a time slot it gets in most places—for a while it was broadcast at 7:00 A.M. *on Sunday* in my area! It's hardly a time when I would be awake watching television!

Another network attempted a show with a similar format, this time on commercial television. It took about five minutes of viewing to register a completely negative reaction in my household. The mistress of ceremonies, the glamorous daughter of a famous movie star, was half the age of the audience for whom the show was intended. All the commercials were oriented toward the young—*not one* included a representative of the audience for whom the show was supposedly intended. And here, too, the time slot was of interest to me. It was televised at 7:30 on a Saturday night. Now, of course, everyone knows that middle-aged people don't go out on Saturday night—we all sit home and long for our younger days of carefree weekends on the town. I do not know if the program is still being aired, and I frankly do not care.

At the White House Mini-Media Conference there was a slight note of hope in another area, though it was just as quickly dashed. After commenting on the fact that broadcast television has rarely acknowledged the existence of senior citizens, much less their needs, a suggestion was made that "cable TV can change all that. In many communities 'public access' channels have been set aside for programs produced by local groups. However, only about a tenth of all cable systems have public access channels, and only a small fraction of these carry programming by and for seniors."

Again the bottom line is money. After making the first optimistic statement, the report concludes, "As channel time increases in value, nonprofit programs may be bumped off." Coming from a very tough New York neighborhood, I loved the last two words, "bumped off." They could not have been more succinct nor more appropriate.

# Advertising and Commercials "We Pause Now for 30 Seconds of Youth"

Now that I am 57 I am allowed by society to be eccentric. Nay, society *demands* that I be eccentric if I am to fit into the mold. Society will, therefore, be happy to know that I am, indeed, quite idiosyncratic. I talk back to commercials.

I talk back to television commercials. I talk back to radio commercials. I even talk back to newspaper advertising that strikes me as stereotypical. I am currently spending my mornings talking back to an executive who does radio commercials for his large corporation and who is busy trying to get me to write to my congressman because the tax laws are unfair to big business. Interestingly enough, I have observed the end result of all this talking back. Not a damn thing seems to happen to change the advertising industry.

If television and its programming are on the "hit list" of the aging group, then the advertising community must certainly be at the head of the class. For some years I was involved in the production of television commercials. I moved away from them because of the frustrations involved in working with advertising people. Much of the copy, the design, the marketing approach, and the supervision in advertising (and thus in the TV-commercial world) is done by the young "geniuses" of the industry. After a recent visit to one of the leading agencies in the country, I was struck once more by the fact that the advertising copy is not only *directed* toward the "Pepsi generation"; it's also *written* by them. Even when the agencies do target the older audiences (at the specific times I'll mention later on), they seem to flounder and miscarry. As Richard H. Davis of the Andrus Gerentology Center puts it, "Advertisers who have their copy prepared by youthful creative geniuses may fail to sell to an older audience they wish to target because of inappropriate techniques employed by those individuals, who do not truly understand that the currently fashionable advertising methods may turn away older audiences."

What are those attitudes? Advertisers are convinced that such things as brand preference and buying habits are well formed by the time we are in our 30s and that they don't change very much as we enter our 40s and 50s. The White House conference reported that, of 147 advertising firms, only 6 *percent* were actually targeting an audience past the age of 35! The figure would be infinitesimal enough if the over-35s were included in the usual range of products: automobiles, travel destinations, food products. But the 6 percent were devoting their efforts almost entirely to denture cleaners, little liver pills, laxatives, pantyhose with tummy control tops (all necessary for that gradual physical breakdown), life insurance, and *coin collecting*. (The latter is to keep us busy during the hours when we're not sleeping or watching commercials on television.)

You don't have to tune in for very long to find the catchword for television advertising (and, to a great extent, the ads in newspapers and magazines). It has five letters that spell "YOUNG," and it is ubiquitous and frequently disturbing. It is not only the beauty products that promise a "different, younger look," or "younger-looking skin," for even in their feeble attempts at change, the copywriters manage to trip over their typewriters. I watched a recent commercial for Camay and heard the phrase, "for a beautiful complexion *at any age!*" I looked up, startled. Where was the word "young"? Was the advertising world changing at last? The women shown first were between 20 and 30. The woman shown on the screen last did look quite attractive, and the announcer intoned, "See how lovely she looks at 41!" The end. Life begins at 40, and ends at 41? And so does beauty? Of course, I talked back to the commercial. To no avail.

Advertisers favor younger women to sell the products, no matter what the category. On the other hand, they consider age an asset in men. The celebrity, of course, is age-irrelevant, since reputation and instant recognizability are factors in choosing the spokesperson. In the world of "voice-overs"—the off-camera actors who sell the product without being seen on the screen—men are chosen between 80 and 90 percent of the time. The advertising industry claims that the choices are based upon "substantial market research and the testing of specific commercials" before they are put on the air.

Now let us look at the *way* in which older people are shown, if they appear at all. As a character in a television commercial increases in age, that character's *physical activity* decreases in direct proportion, and his health problems increase at a rapid rate. In a study done in 1976 the researchers found that 3.2 percent of the characters between the ages of 30 and 40 experienced some sort of health problem, from headaches to minor arthritis. However, as the characters entered their 60s (and up to 70), almost 35 *percent* were complainers of ill health. In the real world, the study concluded, people between 60 and 70 do not experience ten times the number of health problems of any other age group.

The youth culture makes itself still more evident in the implied promise of most commercials—sexual conquest. In every such commercial ever screened by a researcher—and there have been many—the high degree of sexuality involves young and attractive actors. This is no different, I might add, from the advertising that fills the pages of our magazines and newspapers. Just look at the promises of Bermuda and Nassau and all the outer and inner islands. Look carefully at the photographs that accompany the advertising copy. All young. All impossibly attractive. All sexy. *We* are probably back at the hotel sleeping again, or watching Bermudian television.

When we do appear in commercials, the products are either

impersonal or "just right" for our generation. Or else we play the role of the forgetful grandmother or provide an image of the way all us happy people did things "in the good old days."

It is an unchanging part of the pattern and we, again, are the victims. We live in a society that demands that we project a certain image of ourselves when we reach a particular age. Society, in fact, is telling *us* when we are to grow old. And if we have grown old, we have less social value, less economic worth, less feeling of self-worth. The advertising and the commercial messages, ever present in our vast media, are the amplifiers of these precepts. The images, as a result, have the power of commandments. And it is no wonder that the older viewer becomes angry and filled with anxiety.

Interestingly enough, the television commercial field is one place where the pressures we can bring to bear have begun to show some slight effect. The portrayal of older persons as characters has improved somewhat, and more and more messages are being directed toward the middle-aged and the elderly. This can probably be attributed not only to the organizations that have mounted strong protests, but also to the Rip Van Winkles of the ad world who have suddenly discovered a brand-new market. Instead of the "Fountain of Youth," they have belatedly located the "Affluence of Age." Both subjects will be covered in later chapters. But for now, it is time to wander over to our bookshelves and see how well (or poorly) we fare between the covers.

# Our Popular Prose: Balderdash on the Bookshelves

I arrived at New York's Pennsylvania Station on a rainy morning, too early for the train. It is, unfortunately, my destiny to remain a "Type A" personality, one who can never be late for an appointment or a train or plane departure, and one who is impatient with those who are perpetually tardy. Born of a "hyper" mother and nurtured in the field of communications, "on time" translates more easily for me to "too early." But my penchant for promptness allows me ample opportunity to wander, to observe, to lose myself in the surroundings of a new neighborhood while waiting for the designated hour. It was just such a morning and the train to Philadelphia for my meeting with Maggie Kuhn was still more than two hours away. I wandered into a bookshop, though I have never found a book I wanted to buy in an airline or railroad station bookstore. But I do like to wander through them and I revel in looking at the pictures on the covers.

I had become intensely aware by this time of our invisibility and our false images on television and in the world of advertising. I had not realized until then, however, that the problem would extend even into my beloved books. The bookshop, so crowded with easy-to-read, pass-the-time-on-Amtrak paperbacks, was to offer still another view of the youth culture and the invisibility of middle age.

The books in the paperback "sex" section were turned face out so that browsers could not only read the titles, but also could be tempted by the nubile flesh of the half-dressed girls and women who graced the jackets along with the faceless, young, athletic men. And, in case any of us had missed the point of sexuality being only for those under 30, the titles helped set the record straight. *So Young a Bride* next to *Young Girl for Sale* and *Sexy Young Playmate*. A few books down the row, I found *A Bride So Young* and I wondered how much it differed from *So Young a Bride*.

But these "young" titles are accompanied by those marvelous words that tempt us with the story inside (such as it is): Desire, Lust, Ecstasy, Promise, Pleasure, Nymph (or Nymphet), Passion, Horny, and Turning On. Having had my fill of vicarious book-cover sex and not seeing anyone I knew or recognized, I moved on to the romantic novels, published for another trade by firms like Harlequin.

Nothing much is different. The words change somewhat. Instead of Lust, we read Magic and Snowflake and Flame and Stars and Moonlight and Love and Paradise. The jackets still flaunt the lovers, though more fully clothed, yet all of them are *young*. I began to wonder. Where are *we*? Where are the aging faces on the covers of the books? I finally found them.

We are on the *biographies!* We have lived long enough to get our pictures on the covers only if we have achieved something. There *we* were, in all our famous glory—not as half-clothed nymphs cavorting in a *Playboy* bedroom, or standing near a misty castle with Heathcliff coming through the gloom, but in sections of serious reading. Isaac Asimov. Lillian Hellman. Phil Donahue. Albert Einstein. Joan Crawford. Jacob Javits. Luciano Pavarotti.

It was time to hurry so that I could be early at the gate. On my way out of the shop I passed the paperback "sex" section once again and a jacket caught my eye. I laughed, for I had missed it the first time through. The book seemed to leer right back at me as I read the title: *She Liked Them Old*. I mentally thumbed my nose at it and made my way into the cavernous terminal.

The arena of literature and the editorial content of our magazines is but a carbon copy, an instant replay, of the other segments of the media, especially when it comes to the aging. The invisibility and the stereotyping that permeate the television industry and the field of advertising are just as rampant in books, and especially in the literature written for children and young adults, an age when opinions and sensibilities are developed that will be carried through life.

The Council on Interracial Books for Children has been studying the problem and analyzing children's print media for more than 15 years, and though their first target was racism and the stereotyping of blacks and other minorities, they began to uncover a vast array of other stereotypes: about women, about disabled people, about working people—and about the aging.

Acknowledging that the traditional fairy tales and classic children's books presented older people as witches, goblins, and ogres, the council also found that the major problem with contemporary children's books was the same as in the other media: the invisibility of older people in them. Older people, especially sane, useful, active, articulate, sensible, experienced older people, just do not exist. In 1976 they conducted a study of some 700 picture books and found that *almost 600* contained no older characters at all!

The pattern begins to make itself felt again. First invisibility and then less-than-adequate treatment of the characters who do appear. It doesn't change when the literature given to our children is analyzed. Older characters, if they show up at all in *Jane's Trip to the Zoo*, are generally referred to as "old" or "little" or "ancient." I wonder how my friend Alex would feel—all dignified six feet, three of him, a vital man in his 70s—if I were to refer to him as "little old Alex"!

Older characters in children's books also do very little of interest, it seems. They appear as janitors, shopkeepers, elderly grandparents who sit in rocking chairs, grandpa whittling on a piece of wood, grandma smiling—just smiling. How does a youngster reconcile all of this with *you* as a grandparent, if you are one? If children are given the image of the grandmother who stays in the kitchen baking pies, except when she sits in her rocker on the porch, how on earth can they accept the actual grandparent who has just come back from a day of creative work or playing a round of golf, and is dressing to go out to dinner with friends? Their own grandfather, if he tried whittling, might cut his fingers badly, since his job does not require that he know how to handle a knife. And grandmother, in this day and age, may well be a chic, attractive, active woman in her late 40s or early 50s. I smiled when I read an article some time ago stating that everyone accepted the fact that Lillian Carter, the ex-President's mother, was indeed a grand-mother (and a great-grandmother). But Mr. and Mrs. Jimmy Carter are *also* grandparents. So if the children can only think of the rocking chair, how do they reconcile Miss Lillian's flying off to India to visit the people with whom she worked in the Peace Corps when she was in her 60s?

Studies of adolescent literature show much the same pattern, with older characters never in the mainstream of the plots, but merely bit players on the edges—shadow puppets who play out roles unrelated to real life. They are quiet, self-sufficient, never causing any trouble, never "making waves"; underdeveloped people, not so much totally invisible as unimportant. Interestingly enough, the studies of the early literature for adolescents show very much the same patterns of bias, so ageism is not a newly discovered, contemporary phenomenon. It is the awareness that is changing.

Ageism is, of course, omnipresent and our awareness of it is a step forward in trying to change the patterns. Sociologists have found the infestation in every area of the print media. An analysis of more than 2,000 cartoons from a wide range of magazines showed that even in this medium (or especially in this medium), the elderly are treated negatively if at all. Older people appeared only 1.5 percent of the time in the cartoons of the women's magazines, yet I would wager that more than half the readership of those publications is in *our* age group. In the cartoons which did use older characters, most of the themes dealt with sexual or mental dysfunction, political and social conservatism, or oldsters as the butt of a joke or prank.

But even if a cartoon did admit that an elderly person might have sexual feelings, for example, the physical form of that character was totally negative. From time to time *Playboy* magazine has used a sexually oriented, nymphomaniacal elder named Granny. But her physical appearance thwarts the men whom she approaches—sagging breasts, large stomach, very thin legs. In one of the *Playboy* cartoons, Granny stands naked near a group of Western stagecoach bandits and the caption reads, "Honest, lady, we don't *want* to rape anyone!" The cartoons in the slick men's magazines are not the only offending material, however, though they may be vulnerable to attack by the feminists as well as the elderly.

In the studies done on cartoons, the standard magazines were just as guilty in their own way—*Better Homes and Gardens, Ladies' Home Journal,* the *New Yorker, Reader's Digest,* and the *Saturday Evening Post,* to name but a few. My favorite one, though, comes from the *New Yorker.* A middle-aged woman at a bus stop, dressed in the latest of fashion, comments to a dowdy, plainly dressed friend, "I used to be old, too, but it wasn't my cup of tea."

# "Hooray for Hollywood!" A Four-Star Movie Review

There is an interesting thought that occurs when you begin to do research on the media in relation to the subject of aging. Everything written about it in the past still goes on day by day. There's no need to spend weeks in the public library scouring the literature of ancient Roman poets. The phenomenon is a living, breathing perversion of our society, and in each day's newspapers, magazines, television programs, and advertising, the research grows and the monster feeds upon itself to become larger and more apparent.

The motion picture industry is a varied one, and serious films are made by intelligent and well-meaning producers and directors. Though the "pop" movies proliferate for our subteens and teen-agers, all of whom seem to have more money than we do, the small art houses and the independent production companies occasionally try to present a "slice of life." But when Hollywood gets hold of the subject matter for a stereotypical story line, no one can outdo these masters of popular poppycock. My neighborhood has one of those motion picture theaters where, for half the price of the uptown cinemas, the local population can see double-feature cult movies, reruns, classics, and the newly released bombs that have had their three-week run and are doomed to oblivion or to hidden screenings for film students and cinema addicts such as I.

I could not resist this one. The marquee screamed out at me, *Middle Age Crazy!* How could I possibly pass it by, since by that time I was thoroughly steeped in the subject of my writing. I had never heard of the film before. I might hope, after seeing it that beautiful, sunny day when one should have been in the park, that I might never hear of it again. Hollywood did not disappoint me. If ever there was a film that reflected America's self-hate about getting older, it's *Middle Age Crazy*. I wondered, first of all, just what age they might be showing as middle age. They told me right at the beginning.

Bobby Lee (played by Bruce Dern) is celebrating a birthday with his family. It is a difficult time, we find, because he is about to pass a milestone and enter middle age. Bobby Lee is leaving 39 and turning 40. How awful! What a trauma! The entire film is based on the premise that Bobby Lee is having a middle-age crisis of huge proportions.

"Forty," one of the characters states, "that's when the shit hits the fan. That's what happens when you hit 40. You start dreamin' about all those sweet little things you should have been puttin' it to when you were young."

Bobby Lee's wife, Sue Ann (Ann Margret)—the film takes place in Texas so everyone has two first names—tries to keep him confident, happy, and sexually fulfilled, but his mind strays, followed by his "aging" body. At a graduation ceremony for his son (so the boy can leave home to go to college, thus giving them an empty-nest syndrome too), Bobby Lee sees himself making the valedictorian address to the students and their relatives. Wearing cap and gown, he delivers a tirade of self-deprecation denoting the future for which the graduates are destined. "You don't wanna be the future. Give 'em back their silly damn hats and stay 18 for the rest of your lives! The future sucks! You wanna see the future? Look up there at your parents with their big asses and drooping tits! That's the future!" ("T and A" again!)

Well, now Bobby Lee does get some good advice from others in the film, including Sue Ann and his father, who gives him the next big kick in the trousers as an "aging" man. Grandfather, who is 64, advises Bobby Lee, "There's nothin' that makes you feel old like lyin' in a motel and listenin' to someone in the next room screwin'."

In the next scenes Bobby Lee "runs away from home" on business, has an affair with a Dallas Cowboys cheerleader, changes his Oldsmobile for a Porsche and his business suit for cowboy boots and jeans. The sound track blasts out a rock song that warns us, "He's middle-age crazy, tryin' to prove he still can!" (Sonny Throckmorton. Phonogram, Inc., New York.)

There was one marvelous sequence in the film when Bobby Lee decides to throw over his business and his wife for the cheerleader.

Abe Titus, the tycoon who uses Bobby's construction company, is angry over the hero's not showing up for a meeting (since he is ensconced in bed with the cheerleader). Bobby Lee tells him, "I'm not walkin' out. I'm just takin' stock. For all I care, you can take everything and shove it up your conglomerate!" Mentally I applauded, while busily scrawling notes in the darkened theater.

For those readers who follow things like this to their conclusion, let it be said that Sue Ann has her own affair; Bobby Lee comes home after being rejected by Ms. Dallas Cowboy (when he finds her in bed with another man, she reminds him that in her generation there are "no strings attached"), and he ends up in a California hot tub with his wife. Meanwhile the track stridently screams at us once again, "He's middle-aged crazy. Tryin' to prove he still can." The camera pulls back slowly and ends on his Porsche, which he has vowed to trade in for another Oldsmobile.

---

No matter what we do, the media will never be perfect, for none of us are paragons, nor perfect role models for our peers or for the coming generations. Neither are we the only special-interest group to take the media to task for the omissions and the perpetuation of stereotypes. The women in our society have rightly fought the problem, as have the ethnic minorities, and I find that even big business, that sacred cow of our democracy, is beginning to criticize its own treatment by the media.

One of our largest oil companies recently took an ad on the op-ed page of the *New York Times* to complain that the redeeming social values of big business, if any, are not evident in prime-time television. They complained about the characterization of businessmen (as we have about the aging). Two out of three businessmen on television are portrayed as greedy, foolish, or criminal, and half the business they do involves illegal acts. Sound familiar? Television is not only anti-aging. It is also antibusiness. And, without doubt, the business community will fight the image.

And so, then, should we. The first step is awareness. Never underestimate the power of the media to mold opinion and to make us doubt even ourselves. The issue was brilliantly summed up when the ex-governor of New York, Malcolm Wilson, was asked about the public image versus the private man in the case of Nelson Rockefeller. "In today's world the truth is irrelevant," he said, "It's the perception, and the perception comes from the exposure people have to the media."

# Part II
# So Who Are We, Anyway?

Now that we know so many things we are *not*, it is time to move on to discover some of the things that we *are*. For we are a unique generation in a very special kind of society, having shared experiences so alien to the other generations that surround us.

Not only do younger people justifiably profess ignorance when we mention the names of our former movie idols, but they are also insulated by age from the major encounters that shaped our lives, from the Depression through the Big Apple dance craze, World War II, and the Holocaust.

In the same way, we are different from the generation that preceded *us,* and it was we who could not fathom *their* involvement with World War I, Prohibition, and the Black Bottom. Given the changes that take place so rapidly, no one who follows us will ever be quite the same as *we* are, for that is the measure of a changing and dynamic humanity, and it is neither bad nor good. It just *is.*

47

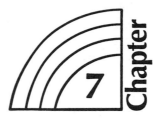

# We Can't All Be Chinese

> *Youth, the curse of the young, the worship of the old.*
>
> > *Fortune cookie served to the author in a Chinese restaurant.*

When the going gets tough, when the awareness overtakes us that life is not always fair, when children talk back to their elders (us), and when newspaper headlines vex us with changes that are violent and unsettling, we can always remind ourselves that the *Chinese* treat *their* patriarchs with veneration and respect. It is comforting to know that somewhere we elders are treated well, with the deference and adoration that we so richly deserve!

It is, perhaps, our own sensitivity toward the personal process of aging that makes us turn toward other cultures and how they treat their aged. I have used the example of the Chinese time and again, even as I have read in the daily newspapers of youth gangs that roam the streets of Chinatown in New York and San Francisco, and of families which are fast disintegrating in the crowded tenements of Hong Kong. It is always better somewhere else; it was always easier at some other time.

And thus I read with a perverse sense of understanding when Colin M. Turnbull writes in *The Mountain People* (Touchstone-Simon & Schuster, 1972) of the treatment of the older people by the members of the Ik tribe in Kenya. He tells of an old man taunted by the children of the village, slapped on the face and knocked over to the accompaniment of laughter and glee. For the Ik, the terrifying treatment of members of the tribe by one another was the result of upending a basically mobile society of hunters and forcing them to become farmers. I wonder what *our* reasons are. And how do other cultures treat their elders?

One thing is certain. In most societies, especially the primitive ones, and at most other times in historical anthropology, the elder was a rare species indeed. Just survival into old age took superhuman effort and a good share of luck. In Elizabethan England, for example, it took the birth of about *nine* children to guarantee that there would be one, or possibly two, survivors past the age of 50. Disease, the pestilence of the Black Plague and smallpox, wiped out a large segment of the population which had survived an appallingly high infant mortality rate. Diet was inadequate (when not poisonous) and wars completed the job that disease had left undone. Even today there are fetid slums around the world where three out of five children die before the age of 5. Given such a ratio, old age might be considered as starting at about 18!

Thus, not only were the elders few in earlier history (as well as in the developing countries today), but these few survivors carried with them, in turn, the knowledge for survival of the entire culture or tribe. Even among the Australian aborigines today, it is the middle-aged men who teach both the boys and the girls of the tribes the crafts, the husbandry, the camp customs, and the tribal lore and rituals.

The outback of Australia is a hostile, waterless, sun-seared desert, so unbearable that I have seen an aborigine stand all day in the shade of a solitary rock, moving with the shadow as the sun traveled overhead, waiting for a passing kangaroo. Should the game appear, the hunter had but one chance to bring it down. I was taught how to throw a boomerang by a middle-aged aborigine, but I have never hit anything with it in my life. Unskilled in the primitive ways, I would starve in the outback.

In such a society the middle-aged men maintain an authority conferred by their age; they are relentless in their discipline of the entire community and in the maintenance of tribal law. It is an elder who is always the leader of the group, knowing more and having had more experience than any other member. At the tribal sessions, it is again the older men who participate while the young men do not join in at all. It is, of course, a male society, and the women do not have the same high status when they enter middle age.

As far back as Babylon and ancient Greece, and even among the Hebrew tribes, it was always the elders, those few survivors, who created a personal gerontocracy, and it was they who most frequently became the prime beneficiaries of the social order. They were the ones who handed down the tribal laws with the admonishment that they were divinely inspired and thus must be followed as they dictated. Ruling councils were, of course, made up only of elders. Even so, I doubt very much that anyone *liked* the idea of growing old.

There is an ancient Japanese poem that says it well. Obviously the poet was not overjoyed with the idea of aging. It was written about 905 A.D.:

> *If only when one heard*
> *That Old Age was coming*
> *One could bolt the door,*
> *Answer "Not at home,"*
> *And refuse to meet him!*

*(Donald Keene, ed. Anthology of Japanese Literature.*
*Translated by Arthur Walley. Grove Press, New York, 1955)*

About ten years ago I set out to produce a television special called *Celebration* and it starred Lorne Greene. It was to be a celebration of *all* stages (sic!) of man's life through five major periods: Birth, Childhood, Adolescence and Betrothal, Marriage, and Old Age. Note if you will that I totally eliminated an entire generation—*us!* At that time I had also become a victim of the myth that we all disappear at the age of 40 or 45, to rest on our plateau until we are ancient. We worked in 15 countries during a single year, including Australia, Turkey, Venezuela, Hong Kong, and Kenya. It was my first strong involvement with the idea that there might, indeed, be significant similarities in the various cultures as well as strongly defined differences.

The aborigines, as I've mentioned, do pass through five very well defined stages of life: childhood, adolescence (the initiation period), early manhood and marriage, the maturity and authority of middle age, and the spirit world of old age. In other tribes, such as the Giriama and the Masai of Kenya, the woman's role in middle age is that of a teacher of the young. She initiates her daughter into womanhood, teaches her about childbirth, knows the remedies for stomachaches, and how to cure the rashes on a baby's skin; she instructs her about teething, herbal medicine, and other remedies passed on by her own parents. For the men of the Masai, however, there is a specific ritual designed to help the warrior shed one role and enter into another capacity in the tribe.

It took many months of preparation and planning before we could get permission to film the Masai ceremonies, and we traveled about 100 miles out of Nairobi to find our contacts and be introduced. Then we spent most of the day being shown the encampment, surrounded by thorn-tree fences; stepping gingerly over the droppings of the cows which live right in the center of the compound, and politely refusing the gourds offered to us. We had been informed that the honey-milk drink was fermented with cow urine and that the teeth must be gritted while drinking so that the flies do not get into the mouth.

The ceremony we filmed is called "passing the fence." When a Masai becomes an elder, he loses his rank as a warrior. Needless to say, the Japanese poem that I have quoted might just as well refer to the Masai, since no warrior likes to give up his role to become an elder, even though the new rank will make him highly respected. The ceremony is in no way connected with the chronological age of the warrior. His time comes when the last of his sons reaches the age of initiation.

For four days the candidate remains isolated from the rest of the tribe while food is brought to him by his wives; only an emergency in the compound or in the prized herd of cows will allow him to leave. Another companion of his during the four days is the honey-wine fermented drink that is present at all Masai ceremonies from the naming of a baby at the age of one to the marriage celebration.

After his stay in the dung-covered hut, the man dons his warrior dress for the last time—the headdress of ostrich feathers, the cape of vulture feathers, and the ankle rings of monkey skins. Armed with his war club, knife, spear, and painted shield, he is ready for his midlife crisis.

The other elders wait for him in his home, still another mud hut topped with cow dung, and the gourds of wine are brought right along with him. The elders chant, "Become an old man. Go, become an old man." And the warrior shouts back at them, "I shall not! I shall not become an old man. No, I shall not!" The fifth time the elders repeat their demand, however, the warrior, now meek and obliging, crosses over into another stage in the Masai culture when he softly replies, "I will go then. I will become an old man." He changes clothing, the warrior's proud adornment left to his sons, and he replaces it with the long, ankle-length dress of the elder. No longer the lion hunter, no longer the fighter and protector of the nomadic village, he is now known as "the father of Gundai" or whatever the name of his son is. For the village, it is an excuse to celebrate with endless gourds of intoxicating honey-milk wine (with flies).

Perhaps our own concepts of the roles of the aged come directly from the rituals of the ancient tribes. Among the Masai the elder "retires" into a life quite different from that of the man he was before. He does not move to the Masai version of Florida or Arizona, but he does a lot of sitting. From that moment on, sitting around the compound all day and smoking their pipes, the elders have a continual conversation about the village, the supernatural, and the current problems. They hear the war stories of retired soldiers. They give advice freely to the young people of the compound, and they mediate and hold councils to see that the ancient Masai ways are continued and the customs are left unchanged. Most of all, they are respected by everyone in the village; I was told that they even become more kindly and friendly to strangers as well as to their own families.

Of course, the treatment of the elder and the entrance into middle life and old age vary from culture to culture, but the fact is that most of the traditional ones are based upon a thinning out of the tribe due to early accident, disease, or living conditions. We may well long for the adulation given the Navajo elder or the Polynesian father and mother (until they came to Hawaii and had to fight desperately to retain their culture), or be wistful about the treatment of aging relatives by the ancient Chinese. But the fact is that no other culture in history has ever had the sheer numbers of older people that we now have and will have increasingly into the twenty-first century. We are not, like the Masai, the exceptional survivors who have entered middle life. Thus our society requires that we look differently at the role of aging.

Our placement in chronologic history cannot change. We cannot, and do not, live in another time, and we cannot change the era in which we are growing older. We would not change our geographic home for the outback in order to be venerated as an aborigine elder, and the affluent, industrial society places us in a totally different role from that of our nomadic cow herder brothers in Kenya. It takes years of learning and the assimilation of both spiritual and practical knowledge for a tribal medicine man to be accepted and respected by the community.

Our doctors graduate from medical school and begin their practice at the age of 27. There was a time when an apprenticeship of five or ten years was required before a young craftsperson or professional entered the world of responsible work. The graduate lawyer or business major today is sought after by large corporations from the day of the commencement exercises, to begin a career at a salary unheard of in our day.

Of course, there was a time when the American household was maintained by the extended family unit and, not being Chinese or Polynesian, we begin to fall back on our idealized memories of the Norman Rockwell view of aging, as immortalized on so many covers of the *Saturday Evening Post*. Whatever happened to the kindly family doctor (who made house calls); the elderly smiling (always smiling) grandmother who took the turkey out of the oven at Thanksgiving; the friendly, ruddy-cheeked general-store keeper with the penny candies behind his glass counter; the primly proper schoolteacher, stern but loving; and the irresistible family dog?

Where, indeed, are the "good old days" that we long for when we find that life changes around us too quickly for us to catch our breaths? Where are the days of yore, when we selectively remember only the good things that happened and a euphoric mist overtakes us to make us long for the stuff of memorabilia? The Broadway shows come back: *Camelot* and *42nd Street* and *Brigadoon*. Those were the days! Or were they?

I wonder how many of us would go back to the labor-intensive days of the last century. The reason grandmother was shown taking the turkey out of the oven was that she rarely left the kitchen. After hauling the water, bathing the kids, preparing breakfast for grandfather and the brood, sewing, cleaning, washing the clothes, and cooking, it's an absolute wonder that she even had the energy to smile for the Norman Rockwell cover! My father would not go back to World War I, I am certain, even though his only stories about that time did not include the three wounds he suffered, but only the good times he had with his youthful comrades. The trenches never existed when he told us his sagas.

There is a delightful book by Otto C. Bettman titled *The Good Old Days They Were Terrible* (Paperback. Random House, 1974) and he forcefully reminds those of us with selective memories that the food eaten by our grandfathers was apt to be ruined by spoilage; street crime was as rampant as it is today; and diseases such as malaria, diphtheria, and intestinal infections took an awful toll of children and adults. Ocean travel for our forebears was in the stinking holds of ships, the steerage in which my own grandparents traveled to this country; and on city streets, the horsecars created a tangle of traffic in dust or mud.

In the Arab cultures there is prevalent an interesting indifference to age. Even the youngest child is referred to as "less than 1," while the "elderly" may be 40, 50, 60, or more. Precise measurements are not critical to their society and, unlike our Western culture, there is no tyranny of time and punctuality. Why, then, in this day and age, must we choose a time to become old? New freedoms have been given to us as well as to the youth of our country.

We no longer have to hurry to "make our mark" by the time we are 30, for as the life span increases and the era of age-irrelevance grows around us, we can take advantage of a second chance and even a third. Our affluence has made us, like the elders of history, a gerontocracy. We control the media, the political arena, the economic structure of America. Why, then, have we succumbed to the myth that it is time to retire from living? At 57, I am still a "pup" in today's society!

The fact is that, by believing all that is told us, we have abdicated the power of our gerontocracy. We forget that the young, who have left our homes in *their* search for freedom, have left us *our* freedom in the process. If the society is more mobile now, and the young leave home not to go down the street to work but to go to San Francisco or Paris to "find themselves" (while we pay air fare to get them there), they also leave *us* unfettered. If they can travel to get away, *we* can travel for our pleasure.

It is time that we surfaced. We may not all be Chinese, but we do not need to be. We do not need the veneration of the young in order to reject our own tribal ceremony, our own rituals that proclaim the coming of age—retirement, withdrawal, invisibility, a halt in our forward movement.

Last night, while reading about the tribal laws of the Navajo, I had a whimsical dream about our own ritual of aging. The last of our children have been initiated into adulthood and are "doing their own thing." I dress in my finest warrior clothing and, carrying my attaché case and business cards, I enter the hut where I am to change my role in our society. I am to become an elder.

However, instead of the other elders being there to judge me and give me the commands, as with my brothers in the Masai, all who sit cross-legged on water beds in the hut are young. They are dressed in their own warrior clothing, designer jeans and T-shirts that proclaim tribal ritual incantations, sayings from the supernatural, and writings of the soothsayers of their generation: "Woodstock Lives," and "We're the Pepsi Generation," and "I Got High in Colorado," and "Sun Your Buns in Venice, California."

The leader is a young girl, barely 15, and her T-shirt reads, "NOW THAT I KNOW EVERYTHING, WHAT DO I DO?" She intones as I enter the hut, "Go. Become an older person." Behind her, the chorus murmurs, "To Florida. To Arizona," and somewhere in the dim half-light of the hut a squeaky voice repeats, "But send money. Send money." Five times the young girl gives her command, "Go. Become an older person," and four times I answer, "No, I shall not!" The fifth time, however, tired of all the repetition, as she utters the magic words, "Go, become an older person," I draw myself up to my full height, my feathers flapping, my monkey skins shining, and I retort, "Go screw yourself!" And with that, I stomp angrily out of the hut.

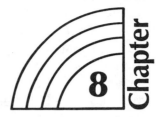

# "Twenty-Three Skiddoo," "Oh, You Kid!" and Other Useful Everyday Phrases (The Language of Us)

> *High thoughts must have high language.*
> Aristophanes:
> Frogs

Some months back, I was one of several guest speakers at a conference in New York. I look forward to these appearances, mostly because I am an inveterate ham who likes to hold forth in front of a captive audience, and partially because I always have a perverse expectation that the luncheon will be a gourmet feast. Of course, I am always disappointed in the hotel fare, generally finding it a cross between an airline meal and a fast-food takeout, though served on elegant china. Nevertheless, I remain optimistic in the face of countless culinary disasters and hours of boring speeches (no doubt including my own).

This particular session dealt with a variety of subjects, including travel, advertising, and communications. The key speaker was a young (about 35) business consultant and, having had my first glass of wine, I sat back expecting to hear a new approach to corporate communications. It didn't take long, possibly a few paragraphs of introduction, and three or four slides, for me to realize with no small feeling of

57

inadequacy that *I did not understand a word he was saying!* This expert on communication was simply not communicating.

Surreptitiously I looked around, thinking that it was I who was lost and that everyone else had just not yet had a glass of wine to dull the senses. I met the eyes of a table partner and he shrugged. I knew I was not alone. Another slide flashed on the screen, the words illuminated in red and green:

> *The disaggregation of a corporation into Natural Businesses is a prerequisite to Strategic Analysis and Formulation. . . .*

My table partner rolled his eyes skyward, we quietly toasted one another with our glasses of wine, and downed the drink quickly, the better to forget what was happening.

We grew up, you and I, in an era of straight talk. When my mother said, "Finish your dinner and do your homework," there was absolutely no doubt in my mind what she meant. The great and the near-great, as well as our families, said exactly what they meant— nothing more, nothing less. Franklin D. Roosevelt told us that we "have nothing to fear but fear itself" and I understood every word. Winston Churchill reported to the British people in the dark days of June 1940, and he said, quite simply, "The news from France is very bad." No gibberish, no gobbledygook. "Bad" meant "bad." The British understood.

But how many of us understood when the crisis at Three Mile Island occurred and someone in the Nuclear Regulatory Commission reported that it was "a failure mode that had never been studied"? Think, if you will, of the panic that might have occurred had Churchill reported the news from France in "high-tech" jargon! As a child, I once had a "failure mode" with my first two-wheeler. My father, poor unsophisticated person that he was, called it an *accident*.

There is no doubt in my mind that one of the greatest areas indicative of the generation gap is that of language. As the new technologies have begun to permeate every sector of our society, the virulence of slipshod and vague abstractions has infected our everyday speech, our schools, our advertising, our business community. In an article in the *New York Times*, Prof. David Ehrenfeld of Rutgers University rightly called it "this pestilence of indirect language." And we, the generations who grew up with straight talk, whose mothers and fathers called it an "icebox" even after it became electric, begin to think that it's *our* fault that we are understanding less of what is being said to us.

Some time ago the Colonial Penn Group ran a series of delightful ads—all of them directed to our generations. One of them, in particular, caught my fancy. It was titled "Do Old People Talk Funny?" and the copy read, in part:

> *We've contended for a long time that young people can and should learn a lot from their elders. Nowhere is this more evident than in language. We think it was George Bernard Shaw who once said that England and America were two great countries divided by the same language. Today, that division has extended to the generations in this country, and probably in England too. It is our view that, as a rule, older people speak more plainly, clearly, and coherently than the younger generation.*

There is a universal quality in the new, ultramodern speech. As it becomes more and more complex, it says less and less. It becomes more abstract, more cleverly phrased, more vague. It is much harder work to be precise. It takes a less fuzzy mind, and if we become too explicit about what we mean, it can be downright dangerous. Dr. Ehrenfeld places a large part of the blame for the new speech patterns at the doorstep of a bureaucracy with too much to hide.

Our generation went to school, we rode in elevators, and some of our grandparents grew up on the farm. In what Richard Mitchell (*Less Than Words Can Say*. Little, Brown & Co., New York, 1979) calls "The Principle of Unnecessary Specification," the little red schoolhouse has become "a venue for learning systems served by a professional infrastructure," and we no longer ride in an elevator, at least not by technical standards. When I recently visited a friend in a tall apartment building, I got to the 15th floor in an "integrated, single-module, vertical transportation system" operated by "an integrated, single-module, transportation system operations engineer"! And the "farm" has given way to "a macro-agricultural environment." No wonder the young people are leaving them to go to the big city (or "urban infrastructure")!

Am I exaggerating? Look around you—words like "macro" and "micro" and "state of the art" and "spiritual actualization." We no longer live our lives—we "function." This trend is ubiquitous and sometimes overwhelming. One of my books won what I might have called "second prize" when I was in a "professional learning infrastructure." However, the new society thinks that I might be terribly disappointed at being second, so the award reads, "First Runner-Up." I no longer live in an apartment. I have "created my own space."

There was a time when I might have looked for a job and the Help Wanted columns would have listed occupations such as "nurse" or "historian" or "sales manager." Some of these archaic job descriptions still exist, of course, but the Help Wanted page becomes even more complicated with the times in which we live. In the Help Wanted columns of our Sunday newspaper, I found an ad that read, "Engineers—Software/Hardware. *We Speak Your Language*." I realized again, just as I did at the luncheon meeting, that not only did they *not* speak *my* language; they were not speaking the language of millions of our generation. There were jobs in "biomass" research, "wafer-fab" engineering, and "microprocessing," one of them requiring knowledge of "MRP theory, MRP software (MAC-PAC, MAPIC, COMSERV-AMAPS), and System 34."

Arlington County, Virginia, recently advertised for an "Urban Revitalization Facilitator" and United Technologies is looking for professionals interested in "shipboard sensor correlation with AN/SYS automatic detection and tracking systems." It transcends the technologies, for the cities have dubbed the people who pick up our garbage every day, "sanitation engineers"! *My* language indeed!

Possibly all this would be quite all right if it were kept within the boundaries of the technological development of our society, as in the sciences and the highly developed electronics and space industries. I am certainly not against technical achievement and progress. I am even willing to give up my Victrola for the latest product in my newspaper ads: "Sonic Holography including a time-delay system with controllable reverberation mix and SL-7 Linear Tracking Turntable, an Autocorrelator system, and a peak-unlimited downward expander." It even has an on-off switch!

But "newspeak" gibberish is everywhere, and when we begin to use our common, ordinary, straightforward language, it is *we* who are accused of "talking funny." A presidential press secretary, caught in a lie, calls his previous statements "inoperative." The perfectly acceptable, old-fashioned term, "togetherness," has become "integrative familial tendencies." The simple, forceful, descriptive word "now" has evolved into "at this point in time." Can you imagine our mothers or fathers saying to us when we were children, "You'd better clean up your room and I mean *at this point in time!*"

Oh, our generation is not entirely innocent by any means. Along the way, many of our peers have contracted the disease of tortured syntax and modern malapropism. Secretary of State Alexander Haig has given the Washington press corps a field day with what has now become known as "Haigese," an almost totally obtuse language. Many of his utterances have become classics. "Theological isolation of a functional objective" is but one. "When we find ourselves in a dialectic fashion at one end of the spectrum" is yet another "Haigism."

There is a classic example of how the language has changed around us, created by the transformations in the relationships of young people in our society. Years ago, when there were intimate relationships developed by the young, many of them were quite innocent by today's standards. The dated language of so many years ago just doesn't hold up for today's social couplings, especially when it is no longer "his place" or "her place" but "their place."

And so the language of an earlier time, descriptive in its simplicity, has given way to confusion and abstraction again. The Colonial Penn ad, "Do Old People Talk Funny?" told a part of the story:

> *Not too long ago, an attractive young lady of impeccable breeding and unusually good manners made passing reference to a social engagement involving one of her "beaus." Her contemporaries in the group looked a little puzzled. Older people present smiled benignly. It was unusual to hear such a young lady use such an old-fashioned word.*
>
> *Later, the younger adults attempted to pinpoint her meaning. Did "beau" mean lover, intimate friend, special companion, roommate, casual acquaintance, or what? They thought it was a funny word to use. The older people thought the word was perfect. It said enough about the relationship. It didn't say too much or tell people more than they wanted, or had a right, to know.*

If you have children who have left home and have taken on the new colorations of cohabitation without marriage, of noncommitment, do you now find it difficult to introduce them to your friends—not because they live together, but because the relationship defies a specific description in today's popular language? "I would like to introduce you to my son and his 'significant other' " or "Meet my daughter and her roommate, George." A famous conductor was reputed to have had a long-time "intimate companion," while a young friend of mine honestly admitted to living with his friend in "sinful cohabitation."

Strangely enough, it is the bureaucrats, so guilty of doubletalk themselves, who have finally come up with a solution to this problem. The Bureau of Census has invented a word that is quite descriptively accurate. Your son's or daughter's live-in partner is merely called a "posslq"—or, in explicit language for us older folks, "person of opposite sex sharing living quarters." And there you are—"I'd like you to meet my son and his posslq."

There is one segment of society in which the new "high-tech" word brokers are having some trouble, however. That group is *us*. They just don't know what to label us and they have been trying desperately to categorize our generations in "newspeak." So far their efforts have been feeble failures. "Middle-aged" is too simple a depiction and even the words "aging" and "elder" belong to our descriptive language more than theirs. We are, indeed, a challenge to them. They've tried "senior citizen" and they've tried to tell us that we are entering our "harvest years" or our "golden years" and that we are getting riper, grayer, or mature.

Unfortunately, these attempts pale when compared with the descriptions they can come up with for schools, elevators, job designations, the old family farm, and the space shuttle program. I wait with great anticipation to see what the young technical wizards come up with that will, once and for all, put us into our semantic places while still reflecting their feelings about those of us who are getting older.

There is no doubt that it will come. One day we will open a newspaper or a magazine and find references to ourselves among all the words that are poisoning direct communication and honesty. We will know it's about us because the article will deal with the "Primogenital Humanoids Commencing Obsolescence."

Who said, "You can't teach an old dog new tricks"?

# It Is Just Possible
# That "Midlife Crisis" Ain't

> *In the middle of the journey of our life, I came to*
> *myself within a dark wood where the straight*
> *way was lost.*
>
> Dante:
> Inferno (1310-20)

$I$ must have been about eight years old when I first became aware of that terribly threatening word, "crisis." In the hushed tones that my mother reserved for matters of grave importance, or for subjects not fit for "the children," she worriedly explained to my father that my three-year-old brother, ill with pneumonia, was at "the crisis." Mind you, it was not *a* crisis. It was *the* crisis, when either the fever, reaching its peak, would drop precipitously or the patient would be in desperate straits. That illness was, indeed, a true crisis for my younger brother and just possibly it was also a crisis for me—a wrenching, helpless emotional experience which stays with me today.

Well, *the* crisis passed and the fever broke. My brother survived beautifully, even before the discovery of penicillin. And—if I can believe the literature, the media, the articles that appear daily—he and I have survived at least two hundred other crises in our lives in order to reach middle age and prepare ourselves for the worst crisis yet to come.

The problem I have is that, given the penchant of Americans and our media to use this word for every change, every stage of progression through life, I fear that I will not even be able to recognize my midlife crisis when it descends upon me! We live in a crisis society. My reading for these past few years leads me to believe that we have a crisis in currency, in health care, in our marriages, in our child-rearing habits, in the kitchen (as well as the bedroom); a crisis in loving, being loved, and being unloved. We have lived through a missile crisis.

Our children are deprogrammed out of religious cults by a process called "crisis counseling." Recently I found that the motion picture industry was also plagued by the disease, as I read an article titled "The Real Crisis in American Films" (as distinguished from the fake crisis). This very morning the newspaper tells me that New York is in the midst of a "vagrant crisis." It stands to reason, then, that *we* were next in line to be noticed. Dr. Bernice Neugarten, with her marvelously fresh view of middle age, wrote in *Prime Time* magazine ("Must Everything Be a Midlife Crisis?" February 1980):

> *The media have discovered adulthood. Gail Sheehy's* Passages, *Roger Gould's* Transformations, *and a dozen other popular books have all accorded adulthood the treatment of high drama, drawing from Erik Ericson's writings, George Vaillant's* Adaptation to Life, *Daniel Levinson's* The Seasons of a Man's Life, *and other studies. Journalists and psychologists make news by describing a "midlife crisis" as if it were the critical turning point between joy and despair, enthusiasm and resignation, mental health and illness. People worry about their midlife crises, apologize if they don't seem to be handling them properly, and fret if they aren't having one.*

A popular stand-up comic recommends that, if you are not having your midlife crisis on schedule, you go immediately to a camp in the Catskill Mountains where experts will induce one for you. the *Wall Street Journal* publishes a cartoon depicting a large group of weeping adults in a living room as the hostess explains, "I thought they'd hit it off. They're all going through their midlife crises." The bookshelves remind us, if other segments of the media have failed: *The Gray Itch* (The Male Metapause Syndrome), *Women of a Certain Age* (The Midlife Search for Self), *The Male Mid-Life Crisis* (Fresh Starts After 40), *The*

*Forty-to-Sixty-Year-Old Male* (A guide for men and the women in their lives . . . to see them through the crises of the Male Middle Years), *The Wonderful Crisis of Middle Age*. After an afternoon in my local bookstore, I became so depressed that I wanted to purchase another book called *Exit House: Choosing Suicide as an Alternative*.

It is a trap. And again we are the victims if we believe everything we read and hear about ourselves. It all seems so logical to us. If the changes through which we live are described as *crises,* it makes it easier for us to accept the fact that we do constantly change, that life is a complex, unpredictable, frequently illogical series of events that do not necessarily take place at predetermined intervals in time.

Certainly there are some crises that are apt to happen more often at certain ages than at others. For example, we are more likely to suffer the death of a parent (or a peer) as we grow older, and Daniel Levinson's "settling down" is more apt to include first marriage and children at 25 rather than 55. Yet 25 percent of all *second* marriages take place after the age of 50! Are not *both* crises example of *normal* change, normal growth, a normal life cycle? The crises of our lives for the most part are as age-irrelevant as the entire society. And though Levinson also declares that "it is not possible to get through middle adulthood (45–60) without having at least a moderate crisis," he does indeed specify critical periods in the lives of subjects in their 20s and 30s. I suggest, then, that too much is being made of our midlife crisis, whether or not we have encountered one so far. The crisis, the event, the change, the transition, the pointing by the fickle finger of fate has less relevance to age than we care to admit in this era of categorizing and putting our lives into neat, well-defined little packages. Look at this list of crises, add your own if you like, and tell me at what age they occur:

> The loss of a job.
> Divorce and legal custody of the children.
> Death of a peer, a parent, a child.
> Change of career.
> Failure or rejection of some significance—the actor who is constantly rejected, the professor refused tenure at a university.
> Severe illness—a young woman who spent three months in a hospital during her freshman year at college because she was allergic to penicillin.
> Catastrophic illness—the breadwinner suddenly found to be ill with cancer, and not covered by major medical insurance.

⚅ Extended unemployment—the hapless, unskilled black or the mother who wants to return to the work force but cannot find a job.

As young people, we thought the crises of our lives were insoluble. The rebellion of the teen-age generation is a crisis for them and for us, else why would drugs and adolescent suicide and teen-age pregnancy be such strong factors in our contemporary catalog of social problems? We may make light of the crises of the young, but if we think back to our own high school days, the first signs of acne before the senior prom were as serious to us then as the empty nest, menopause, or limited retirement income is to us now. One writer even listed "orthodontia" as a crisis of the young!

It cannot take but an instant for the reader to think back to the trauma and the horror of the death of a young peer. I had spent four years in the Army during World War II, and I suppose it was to be expected that one might hear of a friend lost in action or of another friend killed in an airplane accident over Texas while on a training flight—a death especially ironic, since he had survived 75 bombing missions over Germany! But it was wartime and horror stories competed with one another for our attention. Death was a constant companion of life and so many were perishing that the death of a single person paled among so many.

But not too many years later, when I was 31, my best friend, Midge, died of cancer. She was only one year older than I and pregnant at the time. It was Christmas when I got the news and, though I had seen her waste away during the previous year, I could not accept the fact that death would be the end result, certainly not in someone so close, so vital, so gentle, and so very bright. I cried for most of the day and took my car and rode uptown to visit her husband, roundly cursed by taxi drivers for my erratic behavior on the road. And each Christmas, even to this day, depression sets in and it suddenly occurs to me that I am still torn; that I still miss her so many years later.

Of course it was a crisis. And many have occurred since then. I am stating, as strongly as I can, that crises can come at any time and that they are not predictable, like preordained transitions that take place at a particular stage. Neither am I stating that crises do *not* occur during midlife. I am merely making a semantic demand that we call a crisis a crisis when it is, indeed, a crisis, while resisting the temptation to label each wind of change as a hurricane. As my friend Frankie says,

"They don't even let you have one bad day. Just try to have one bad day and they call it a crisis."

I was speaking to a middle-aged friend about her feelings at this time in her life, and the description of a friend of hers is a case in point:

> *This is a woman who is, first of all, very heavy, so she's got a lot of physical things against her. About four or five years ago when her husband, a brilliant engineer, moved out to live with his younger secretary, she didn't have any money problems. She even started college, finished it, and went on for her degree in business administration. She was, effectively, alone, and she got kind of used to that.*
>
> *Then her husband contracted cancer and he came home to her to die! He died within a month. She actually took him in when he came back. She was furious at him, but she took him in. He left her well off, with about a quarter of a million dollars.*

I asked what had happened to his young secretary.

> *I don't know. I suppose she gave him up when he contracted cancer. It was quite a scene—a heavy afternoon when my friend and I went to clear out the apartment that her husband had shared with his secretary. Well, it now turns out that my friend's lawyer has absconded with most of the money her husband left her. Within the year, her father died of cancer and a brother who lived in the Caribbean area died of a brain hemorrhage, leaving her without any support system at all. All within a year. What would you call this?*

Well, I would call it a *crisis!* But the example cannot be used to proclaim the coming of middle-age crisis for an entire generation. There is no common pattern of change, nor is there a consistency of life style, adult conflict, or entrance and exit through rigidly fixed stages. Gail Sheehy labels her ten-year passages, for example, as "The Trying Twenties" or "Passage to the Thirties," and Levinson says of a writer in his early 30s that "by this time . . . it was *late* to develop his talents." (Italics mine.) Dr. Neugarten answers these authors by stating, first of all, that the media coverage of middle age is based on too little evidence (Levinson on only 40 men and Vaillant on 95 Harvard grads). She adds:

*Choices and dilemmas do not sprout forth at ten-year intervals and decisions are not made and then left behind as if they were merely beads on a chain.*

*It was reasonable to describe life as a set of discrete stages when most people followed the same rules, when major events occurred at predictable ages. People have long been able to tell the 'right age' for marriage, the first child, the last child, career achievement, retirement, death. In the last two decades, however, chronological age has moved out of sync with these marking events. Our biological time clocks have changed.*

She explains further that the onset of puberty is earlier than it has ever been, menopause arrives later for women, there are new life styles in work and career orientation, and people are living into old age as healthier, more active adults. When the children leave home, the parents now find the freedom to pursue a range of new activities and an expansion of their vital life style.

I look at Levinson's description of the writer in his 30s and laugh as I look back on the publication of my *first* book when I was 54 and four subsequent books that followed. I am amazed at the number of my friends who are starting new lives, new vocations, new careers in their 50s and well into their 60s, and I read with some sense of vicarious pride that Dr. Neugarten's own husband, Fritz, started a new business at the age of 65!

The theory of "age-irrelevance" is not without its detractors, however. In spite of a society that is changing around them, some sociologists and other scholars are throwing up their hands in horror at the very thought that we may be entering a new era of aging. Using the term "life-span specialists" (a contemporary designation which might well have gone into the previous chapter), they proclaim that the social order will be destroyed if we do not have age norms as an "anchor."

One sociologist even goes so far as to state that an age-irrelevant society is a rudderless one. A gerontologist terms the theory preposterous. After all, if we can sell the idea successfully, where will all the myths and stereotypes go? And what will happen to our middle-age crisis if it doesn't appear on time? If, as still another gerontologist contends, age-irrelevancy will encourage the old to try to stay young, thereby denying them the dignity of old age, I must ask if *dignity* is a private monopoly of the elderly.

It is terribly unfair to our generations to characterize our problems and crises as indicative of our age rather than point out that much of what we experience during the middle years is quite normal and very much to be expected. As with any popular subject—sex, diets, positive thinking, religion—the bandwagon of middle-age crisis has triggered its own set of self-fulfilling stereotypes. Certainly, middle age brings its own set of problems, its own specific and individual changes, and even some emotional difficulties. But, in fact, not even a majority of our generations suffer the personal conflicts, identity crises, career upheavals, or family difficulties that might characterize a good, healthy midlife crisis. The Chinese, in all their wisdom, seem to have found the truth again, for the Chinese word for crisis is composed of two characters—one signifies danger; the other represents *opportunity*.

The word "crisis" becomes superficial and meaningless when it is tied to a life style of normality, repeated over and over again in millions of contemporary family situations. I will discuss this more in later chapters, but it is not a crisis when the children finally leave home, and it is perfectly normal when three generations of family members are living their own active and fulfilling lives. As we age, we begin to plan for retirement, accepting the fact that we will (or will not) give up our work to pursue other activities. And though we try not to dwell on it, the aged do accept death as a part of life.

On the other hand, if we were so ridden with middle-age crises, our lives so distorted by the emotional upheaval of passing a particular milestone, it seems to me that we would be filling the mental hospitals and the psychiatrists' offices to overflowing. In actuality, the admission of patients to mental hospitals grows rapidly up to the age of about 34, then *drops* gradually through middle age, to rise again after age 65. If we were to investigate the statistics of extremes, the suicide rate for teen-agers is far higher than that of our age group.

Some time ago psychologist Douglas Bray and his colleague Ann Howard did a 20-year study of more than 400 employees of the Bell System. It dealt with career success and life satisfaction of middle-aged managers and one of its most interesting conclusions was that only 22 percent of the subjects were undergoing what might be considered a midlife crisis. This means that the great majority were *not*.

The authors of the report are not without a sense of humor. Since so much attention was being paid to crisis in middle life by psychologists, psychiatrists, and sociologists, they also came to the conclusion that "the middle-aged male was threatening to replace the white rat and the college sophomore as the dominant research subject in psychology."

Up to this point you have probably noticed an overwhelming balance in favor of the *men* of our age group. Though they offer various forms of apology for omitting more than half the population, researchers and authors have, until this time, concerned themselves almost wholly with men. Daniel Levinson did not have the funds to pursue a thorough and balanced study of both sexes in *The Seasons of a Man's Life*. Vaillant studied *male* Harvard grads because there were only male Harvard grads at that time. When Bray and Howard began their research with Bell System middle-level managers, well over 20 years ago, almost all (if not all) in that category were, of course, men.

The reports reflect both the attitudes and the demographics of our society—male-oriented, the woman at home taking care of the kids. If a woman played any role in the job market, she was generally paid less than men (and still is in most cases); she was not eligible for equal pension rights, she sublimated her professional choice to the location of her husband's job, and the potential of top management was denied her (and still is, for the most part). To top it off, she was always expected to look "young."

Are women, then, not allowed to have their midlife crises, even in fantasy? If, as the studies show, women have more stressful life experiences than men, if differences between *the sexes* are more significant than differences between young and old of each sex in terms of economics, emotional stress, and society's demands—not to mention fulfillment—then it stands to reason that women, too, should be entitled to feel the "panic" of middle age.

We do not, in fact, need the studies to tell us that widowhood, divorce, reentry into a job market that was so very different 20 years ago when the woman left it to raise a family, and a society that demands that we look younger than we have a right to are all factors that lead to a reassessment and a reevaluation during midlife. The rising awareness of women in our society, the political organizations that fight for equal rights for the aging as well as for women, the struggle to right a thousand wrongs over a period of centuries—these subjects will be covered in Chapter 20. It is difficult enough to face the *realities* of the conflict without the added burden of the myths. And it is those myths with which I am most concerned. In order to have a real, honest-to-goodness midlife crisis, there are certain parameters that hold true for women as well as for men.

It is the unexpected event—or the expected event that happens at an unexpected time—that creates the need for an explanation of what we are going through. Panic, transition, crisis, adaptation, coping, stress. The young woman entering puberty *anticipates* the beginning of menstruation. It is not a crisis, certainly. Wanted pregnancy creates a normal and mostly happy transition; unwanted, it can be a disaster, no matter at what age it occurs. The death of a child upsets the rhythms and tranquility of a life cycle much much more than the death of an aged parent or grandparent. Dr. Neugarten calls it "the psychology of timing" and indeed it is. Widowhood at an early age, or sudden widowhood at any age, can be a critical shock, followed by a painful readjustment in a society that demeans widows and singles them out for unequal treatment and loss of status. Nevertheless, as we age, there is a more realistic, underlying perception that widowhood may well happen in our 60s or 70s. Looking around us, we know that many of our friends have been recently widowed. Death, then, may come as a shock, certainly, but the term "crisis" may well not apply.

But it is in the area of woman's sexuality that the male-dominated society has created the most myths, though many of them are being broken down one by one. It is not only that *women* are changing so much. It is possibly that the *society* is being made aware that much of what we have heard and read is pure fantasy. Researchers (bless them) are even discovering that the Victorian woman enjoyed sex, though her demeanor denied everything.

We know, of course, that women are hysterical. Even my mother perpetuated that myth. After all, the word "hysterectomy" comes from the Greek word *hystera* (uterus). Even your doctor believes it! The myths have built up through the centuries and women (as well as men) have had their own strong self-doubts, feeling that if society keeps saying it, it must be true. We all try to live up to other people's expectations, and in this area we are no different than when we were 20 years old. Which brings me, in turn, to the climacteric, or menopause.

I remember my grandmother, then my mother, whispering about "change of life." The flushes; the end of fertility, femininity, sexuality, attractiveness, and vitality. In other words, the end. The worst possible thing that could happen as a woman grew older.

There is no doubt that hormonal changes take place, and with them many psychological ones, but if we believe the women who have written on the subject and the interviews conducted with hundreds of women, the onset of the climacteric is but another event in the gradual growth pattern of the female adult.

Keep in mind that medical literature usually is based upon studies of disease. As a result, we cannot generalize from the findings to include the majority of the population. Certainly, some 75 percent of all women who reach menopause experience disturbance or discomfort, but only a very small percentage visit their doctors for treatment. In a survey conducted by Dr. Neugarten, with 100 normal women between the ages of 43 and 53, only 4 of the women stated that menopause was their major concern. Over 50 percent, however, declared that "losing your husband" would be their greatest worry.

In addition, over 65 percent maintained that there was no change in their sexuality after menopause. And even many of those who thought there was a change felt that sexual relations had become more pleasurable, because *the fear of pregnancy was no longer there.*

A great number of writers have zeroed in on another phenomenon—the "male menopause"—but even here the symptoms of depression and fatigue and the reassessment of life style, job, and family generally have their roots in psychological and job-oriented situations rather than in hormonal changes. This, too, as life expectancy increases, is a normal effect. The term "male menopause" will stay with us, however, because it makes for another gold mine of articles in popular magazines.

When I was a child, I remember crying bitterly at the "trials and tribulations" of a peer of mine as he starred with Wallace Beery in a motion picture called *The Champ*. The child actor was Jackie Cooper and, when he was eight, his weekly salary was $1,500! A few weeks ago I noticed an article in the entertainment section of our newspaper and the headline read, "Cooper: a Star at 8, but Happier at 58."

Briefly, he was nominated for an Academy Award at the age of 8; at 18, he was Joan Crawford's lover. By the time he had reached 28, he was washed-up in the motion picture industry, a victim of Hollywood's star-eating system. He had been divorced twice and, by the age of 38, had again become a star, this time on television. At 58, he is a successful television director and he is quoted as having said, "I am having fun, more fun than I've ever had in my life!"

I suppose that the story that affected me most was Cooper's description of how they made him cry for the cameras. His grandmother would drag his pet dog off the set, where they would "shoot" the poor animal. His life as a child and a young adult was far from happy, yet my mother wanted me to "be like Jackie Cooper."

It is ironic because so much is attributed to youth and its potential. Daniel Levinson calls it, "The Dream of Youth," and yet this 58-year-old actor-director is just beginning to realize his own dream of fulfillment and happiness. And he is not alone. So many of us nurture dreams that we could not fulfill in our youth because of economics, marriage, children, illness, or just plain immaturity and lack of experience. It is terribly unfortunate that so many of us think of adulthood, especially these vital years, as a time of stagnation, punctuated by the trauma of midlife crisis. How sad it is that we believe this fantasy.

Eda LeShan, in her book *The Wonderful Crisis of Middle Age* (David McKay & Co., New York, 1973), calls us "a very tired generation" and she glories in the flower children and their revolutionary spirit of the '60s. Ironically, two years later, right before publication, she wrote an addendum as she discovered that these young vital social insurgents had a bad case of malaise, indolence, and stagnation. In addition, many of them—bored with "doing their own thing"—were moving back into the homes of their parents!

No, we are not a tired generation. My grandfather's generation was tired, mostly because they worked so hard physically to give us what they thought we deserved. The younger people of today are more tired than we, even before they have found something to be tired from. *We,* in turn, are in a time of change and of growth. The demographics are changing and it is we who are growing most rapidly in that change. Our mobility is changing, as is the technology. Our careers, income, family life, politics, and time for leisure will make for an even faster rate of change in our lives than ever before. Tired? Who has time to be tired?

It is normal and quite natural to ask questions as we progress in our lives. It is reasonable to query, "Why me?" when life seems to strike us out. But most of what we experience is all a part of normality, a natural result of change and growth. My friend Carol, over luncheon one afternoon, put it well:

> *Why is it that you expect that at some time in your life everything will go smoothly? You will have a status, finances will be secure, and your personal life will smooth out. Why do you expect that it will happen—but it doesn't?*

Jonathan Swift might have answered her by saying, "There is nothing in this world constant, but inconstancy." I feel that part of living is solving problems, that there must be some challenge in order to create change. As Gail Sheehy put it so well in *Passages,* "If we don't change, we don't grow. If we don't grow, we are not really living."

What we too often call "crisis" is merely growth.

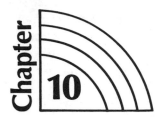

# 10

# The Empty Nest,
# the Bulging Nest,
# and the Boomerang Syndrome

> *For time will teach them soon the truth, There
> are no birds in last year's nest!*
>
> > *Longfellow:*
> > "It Is Not Always May"

Imagine, if you will, another time. You are about to leave your
parents' home, possibly forever. It is a very special time in your life and
in theirs, for you are the last of the children to make your way into the
world. Possibly you have just gotten married, or you are leaving home
to do what passed for "your own thing" in that more naive era. Or
perhaps it is just the four years of college that lie ahead. Whatever the
reason, the secure nest will soon be empty, except for two adults who
have had little time alone together through their 20 or 30 years of
marriage.

You are gone and the first visitor to knock on the door of the
little house, the sounds filling the now empty rooms, is a sociologist
who is taking a survey on what has been discovered as a *new* crisis in
middle life, "the empty-nest syndrome." Breathlessly he or she asks,
"How do you feel about your last child leaving home?"

Think for a moment about how that question might have been

taken by your parents, and especially by your mother. For more than 20 years, she has been conditioned to accept marriage, homemaking, and the rearing of her children as the main function and purpose of her life. To be called a "good mother" is the accolade that she accepts most easily, while sublimating all her frustrations, her dreams, her personal goals. When you left her home, she certainly felt that she might miss you somewhat, since she rather liked you as a person. But deep down, under all the platitudes and the social acceptance of the role model, she has begun to feel a sense of relief and a freedom from bondage. The researcher asks the question again: "How do you feel?"

If she answers truthfully and tells not only of her sadness, but of her relief and the newly found sense of joy bubbling up somewhere in her psyche, she is admitting that she was not that good a mother after all, or worse, that she did not love you. How could she possibly even imply all that to a stranger? The guilt would be too much to bear afterward. Therefore, she tells the sociologist what she thinks she *should* say. After all, this was not a time when women gave vent to their honest feelings, nor a time when a more liberated society accepts such feelings. In the atmosphere of our parents' generation, your mother would be encouraged to dissemble, to bury the feelings of freedom while giving vent to the sense of despair and loneliness that accompanied your going out the door. She would promptly be marked down by the researcher as having a chronic case of "empty-nest syndrome."

This is not by any means farfetched, for out of the distorted studies of the generations right through the 1950s has come one of the most damaging myths about middle age. It is, probably, even more a lie than a myth and it has been especially demeaning and destructive to women in particular.

I wonder why it took so long to discover that women might welcome the end of mothering and see it as a time of liberation. The contemporary surveys, conducted now that people are not afraid to speak their inner feelings, have begun to find that women do *not* suffer unduly when the nest empties and the fledglings have flown off. In one recent study of 160 middle-aged women with an average age of 46, Lillian Rubin of the Institute for the Study of Social Change (University of California at Berkeley) found only *one* who was suffering from the classic symptoms of the empty-nest syndrome! Many were, indeed, ambivalent about their feelings, but almost all greeted the event with a strong sense of relief.

If anything, it is the *fathers* who are more vulnerable to the change in family status, especially those who feel neglected by their wives or who have worked long and tiring hours in pursuit of status and career. Thinking that they can at last spend more time with the growing children, they find instead that the home situation has radically changed. The stereo no longer blares the records of Springsteen and Chicago; they have been replaced by the wife's collection of Bach and Vivaldi. How many *fathers* of our generation have insisted, for reasons of their own, that their children attend a college close to home, while the mothers deeply felt that school on the North Slope of Alaska might be a good educational beginning?

My friend Dee wrote me a long, deeply personal letter. It was his answer to my questions about this strange malady, so much a part of the crisis literature. "In previous generations, people tended to act the way they were expected to act," he wrote. "People of middle age were supposed to act in a particular way. So they did. Consider the European widow dressed in black. She looks old and ugly and plain and alone and stalwart and not full of joy. She probably became like that because everyone wanted it that way. Her children would be ashamed and concerned and grieved if she didn't. Today, most people in America have a lot of options. We can choose *where* we want to be, and we do. And with whom. It's not just an economic choice. There's also a big change in *perception*. People don't have to look old. Or act old. Or think poor."

Friends like Dee have been important to me in this search for a true picture of this stage in our lives. Having no children of my own, I was particularly interested to find out how *they* felt about the empty nest, since all of them were losing children to the cruel world or their offspring had already sprung. How could I know, after all, that the earlier studies were not correct and the newer ones were equally fallacious or inaccurate? No child of mine had ever left the house, never to return. Dee's children had been gone only a short time when he wrote.

"We had a baby 10½ months after the wedding, so we are now, for the first time, going to be 'just a couple.' It's not good, or bad. Just different from all we've known together. We've been excited and anticipatory about the empty nest. . . . We've just begun to experience our new roles. So far, we are going out a lot more—perhaps three nights a week. Eleanor has already changed her reading habits. She always read a lot, almost every day since our marriage. But in the past she read Regency romances, history stuff, and other escapist literature. In recent weeks, however, she has been reading a series of classics like Jane Austen and she has begun Barbara Tuchman's *A Distant Mirror*. Somehow this suggests to me that she has enough stamina or emotion or leftover intelligence to invest, by choice, in something of substance. This, after years of reading only for relaxation and escape."

The reaction is not unusual. Mothers return to college as matriculated degree students, either to continue an education truncated by pregnancy and childbirth or just for the sheer joy of being with other adults in a process of learning and not having to lower her intelligence standards to that of a three-year-old or a teen-ager. Others have returned to the job market, either to continue a career or to find a new challenge outside the kitchen and the car pool.

There are marvelous stories about newly liberated parents changing the entire décor of the house after the children have left. One couple turned a children's wing into an office and hobby shop, much to the chagrin of their progeny when they returned for the holidays, to find that they had been dispossessed in the name of liberation. Another reported with relief that she can now sit in the living room and have a conversation with another adult without having a teen-ager sitting and glaring at them. If the loss is a trauma, it is only transient as new life styles begin to emerge and new options materialize. Here are some examples that surfaced during my interviews with friends.

Time for quiet, candle-lit dinners at home or in a restaurant, alone or with friends. Time to enjoy two in a house with more time for self-indulgence. Time to say goodbye to the youth collectives that camped in the living room. Time to welcome the kids when they come home for Christmas and to admit that it's a joy to see them go again. Time to pursue the hobby that always seemed to elude you. Time to play tennis because you want to rather than because it serves as an escape from the responsibilities of the children. Time to think quietly. Time to be what you always thought you might become. Time to be yourself.

My friend Dee writes, "I'm glad for the new times. I don't feel: 'Is that all there is?' It's just the *past* in a process so gradual that it never occurred in one moment of time. When the boys call long distance, it's nice. But it's not wonderful. It's not like those warm-all-over TV commercials for long distance telephone. I find that days go by when I don't think of them at all. Eleanor acknowledges the same experience, even though she is involved more in sending packages and forwarding their mail to them.

"Our kids are nice. I like them. I'm pleased with them. Each is different from his parents and different from what I thought he was or would grow up to be. I'm glad I did it. I'm pleased I don't have to do it any more!"

On a walk through our island the other day, I came across Emily in her garden. She is on the edge of the empty nest, while Dee has already said goodbye to his children. Her daughter is away at college and the son will leave within a year. "At certain times," she said, "I talk a good game and I say, 'I can't wait for them to go'—but by the time they're both gone, I'll miss them. I don't know what it will be like, but I'm looking forward to it. I'm looking forward to being my own person. I'm looking forward to not having to come home to cook dinner. I'm looking forward to having much more mobility."

She looked up from her garden, determined to be the pragmatist, and she smiled. "I guarantee that when it comes to the holidays, my *neighbor's* daughter will come home and mine won't." I asked her if that disturbed her and her eyes sparkled. "Of course it does," she retorted, *"Who's going to help me cook?"*

# The Bulging Nest

If we have settled the "crisis" of the empty nest, you may be certain that something will replace it quickly. Times have changed so rapidly that it is no longer required that we deny our sense of freedom when the children leave. In fact, many of us admit to anxiously awaiting their exit. *What happens if they don't want to go?* What happens if we buy them an airline ticket to Alaska if we live in New York; New York if we live in Alaska, pack their clothing, open the front door—and they won't leave home? *This* is a crisis!

Ann Landers, the columnist, once advised a parent signed "Hopefully Desperate" to "throw the bum out" when a letter was written to her describing the plight of one family. The mother wrote of a 22-year-old son whom she had tried to evict without success. The young man was in debt, paid nothing for his room and board, lived like a vagrant, kept his room like a pigsty, stole from his father and brothers, and, to top it off, wrote rubber checks. To make matters even worse, the mother complained, "All I can do is refuse to accept his collect calls. But mostly he doesn't call collect. He is *here!*"

Ms. Landers answered the plea with a citation of U.S. and Canadian law that allows a parent to institute a civil or criminal suit for *trespassing* once the child has reached majority. A friend of mine, not so hostile as that toward her 25-year-old son, wailed about the *bulging* nest in her own home. Things were just too comfortable there for the young man ever to consider leaving. The nest would not only *not* be empty, but it seemed destined to be distended forever.

My friend claimed that she had tried everything. "Every night," she said, "I move his bed closer and closer to the front door. But he doesn't take the hint!" I, myself, have sent her the item written by Ann Landers, but other than that, this is one time that I mentally give thanks for not having had any children! I seriously wonder if I, as a father, would have had the courage to "throw the bum out!"

# The Boomerang Syndrome or the Refilled Nest

It comes with a knock on the door or a long-distance telephone call (collect). The life in San Francisco is not quite what it was supposed to be. "Doing your own thing" required sharing the apartment with California's best cockroaches. The trip through Europe to "find himself" included losing his cash to a pickpocket, misplacing his airline ticket, and deciding that he might want to bring his sleeping bag and his new sleeping companion back to your house "for a while."

The economics of the world is too much for the young, newly marrieds to handle, especially since the baby was born and they'd like to save some money to buy a new house at today's astronomical prices. One young couple, interviewed by a reporter, just couldn't save enough unless they gave up their large apartment that had an artist's studio for the wife, dinner out four times a week, and the personal computer just purchased by the husband. So they went "home" to live with their parents until they could straighten out their finances!

The expectations of our younger people are dashed rather easily, it seems. They were brought up (by us) in an era of affluence, with minimal problems of growth and the high hopes that accompany our catering to a generation that "deserved" everything and was rightly labeled with the word, "ME." The very fact that a slight and shallow magazine called *Self* is such a huge success is a tribute to the thinking of the children now reentering the nest in ever-increasing numbers, unable to cope not only with the economics of the world, but with the unfinished business of their emotional growth.

I am not pointing to our generations as paragons of balance, by any means. In our day, when we finally left home we expected much, much less. We settled on a job, any kind of job, even if it were menial and tedious. Perhaps that was a flaw in our personalities. But we expected to struggle and we expected to build our lives bit by bit. The "personal computer" came after the marriage, after the kids, after the career—if it came at all. But the important thing about this new boomerang syndrome is that it strongly tells us that there is no statute of limitations on parenting. You have emptied the nest. Your freedom— your richly deserved freedom—is yours at last, and suddenly you are once again parents, but with extreme differences this time around.

While they were gone, the children developed their own life styles and habits, sometimes affected by the partner with whom they had chosen to live (whether at their house or yours). The returning son is discouraged with the job market, the daughter is just taking up "temporary residence" in your home. The dinners you served when they were growing up are not quite right now, because "you don't know anything about nutrition," and your son George is now a vegetarian. Alice's boyfriend didn't give a damn whether or not she made the bed or cleaned up when they were together in their apartment, but for some reason *you* seem to care. You actually get to like her boyfriend better than you ever liked her (for he has moved right in with her). The problem of a son or a daughter returning to a home where there has been remarriage or divorce is even more severe. The return, for whatever reason, may turn the home into a battleground. And privacy is lost on both sides.

Other than turning the welcome mat upside down when they arrive, the solutions vary. Some parents totally avoid having to face the boomerang by giving up the spacious, four-bedroom house and moving into a small downtown apartment without a guest room, just as soon as the children leave home for the first time. In addition there is an invisible, but strongly worded, sign over the front door that reads, "No Sleeping Bags Allowed."

Others have divided the house into separate living quarters with several common rooms. Still others have begun to achieve some success in this new extended family situation by making use of its positive aspects and the unexpected benefits that can go along with the difficulties. However, my own feeling, after speaking to families who have had to readjust their lives, and after reading many reports on this new phenomenon, is that the advantages are heavily weighted in favor of the young (again).

The economic regrouping and the feeling of inability to cope is strongest in our children and, if they come home to live with us, it is *we* who are helping *them* to adjust to *their* vicissitudes of life. For them it is a chance to "find themselves" yet again, to change direction, or to pursue a new career. If they are a couple and they have children, it is they who benefit from our free baby-sitting, and it is they who can now save for the dream home that we, as parents, struggled to acquire on our own some years back.

For us, there is the possibly renewed feeling of being needed again, for whatever pragmatic reasons. Possibly there is also a challenge and a sense of rejuvenation in the new living arrangements.

But all sides report that it is not easy. For those of us who have welcomed the empty nest, only to find that it is filled once again, the emotional shock can be severe and the sense of anger that we feel is quite natural. It may be difficult, if not impossible, to turn down the request of a child to return home again, but if it happens, the "ground rules" should be laid down firmly and at once. It is, after all, *your* home they are coming back to. The chores of cleaning up after dinner, taking out the garbage, or walking the dog late at night in the rain should be clearly designated or the situation can disintegrate into chaos. You, in turn, may want to think about your demands that your grown daughter be back in the house before midnight, now that she is turning 30. It takes maturity of outlook on both sides to make it work.

Psychiatrists, sociologists, and marriage counselors are watching this new phenomenon closely to see how it all turns out. Anything that replaces the myth of the empty nest will be welcome, you can be sure!

# A Brief Postscript

There is a new extreme surfacing in the family relationships of our generations and, though I smiled when I first heard of it, I am not so sure that it is not a good idea. It is called "benevolent disinheritance." Many parents feel that they have amply provided for their offspring during the 20 or 30 years that it took to raise them, nurture them, send them through college, and provide loans for their first business ventures. Their children are financially secure, do not need their help any longer, and are quite independent.

As a result, there is a growing trend to cut the children out of the last will and testament. A large number of children have been out of contact with their parents for years. In many cases, no close relationship even exists outside of blood. On the other hand, in their later lives, the parents discover that friends and neighbors are more in need of their money than their children are. Thus the disinheritance, and the accompanying outcry of the children left at poverty's door along with their personal computers. It is the same shriek of pain that we sometimes hear from our children if we remarry when we are widowed or divorced. Many presume that the new spouse is obviously out for our money!

We are, of course, entitled to lead our own lives, whether in our empty nests or with our own "posslq," at whatever stage of our growth and regardless of the complaints of our children. We are entitled to do as we please, go where we please, and live where we please. We are also entitled to do with our savings and our pensions exactly what we please. And so the idea of "benevolent disinheritance" strikes a chord in my perverse sense of humor. This in turn reminds me of a famous George M. Cohan song, "Always Leave Them Laughing When You Say Goodbye!"

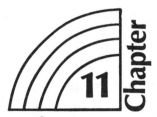

11

# The Sexy Sexagenarian (Everything We Wanted to Know about Sex, We Knew a Long Time Ago)

> *I'm Not a Dirty Old Man—*
> *I'm a Sexy Senior Citizen!*
> *Bumper sticker seen in Florida*

The New York taxi driver, always the philosopher of unsolicited trivia, made his way slowly through the crawl of midtown traffic. I sat back, resigned to a long trip, sorry that I had not walked the short distance, while he droned on, covering the present administration in Washington, the past mayoralty of John Lindsay, the influx of undesirables into the city, and, finally, the current news story being covered with the thoroughness of World War II. A famous diet doctor had been shot four times by his paramour and the murder trial was yielding ample subject matter for feminists, people on diets, the millions who had read his book, and New York taxi drivers. For most of the stop-and-go trip I barely listened to the monologue, but one comment made me sit up and take heed, for I was, naturally, right in the middle of my research for this book.

"What the hell," he screamed over the blaring din of horns, "He   83 was no angel. He was screwing everything that moved. I don't even know how he could do it. He was *70 years old!*"

Not too many weeks after the incident, while deciding whether to attack what follows with humor, wit, and sarcasm—or with the anger that I had begun to feel at the perception of older people (including us middle-aged) as asexual, nonsexual, or sexually expired, much like *Tyrannosaurus rex*—some contemporary friends and I were discussing a woman of about 52. And once again I heard it and wondered why I had not been aware of it before—even among our peer groups.

The woman's daughter (she was 26) was complaining because her mother had rented a summer house with some younger people and had become a "swinger." The daughter was, of course, distraught. Her mother, in her words, had gone into her *second childhood*. My contemporaries seemed to agree. This woman's mother was not *acting her age*.

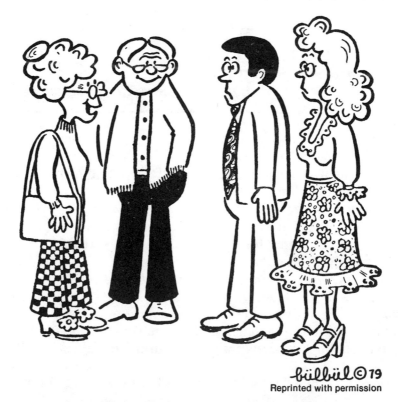

bülbül © 79
Reprinted with permission

NO SON, CHARLES AND I ARE NOT JUST FRIENDS . . . WE'RE LOVERS.

The Roman sage Publilius Syrus wrote, "It is natural for a young man to love, but a crime for an old one." It took some centuries for an answer to be written (in 1972) by Simone de Beauvoir, and it was long overdue:

> *If old people show the same desires, the same feelings, the same requirements as the young, the world looks upon them with disgust; in them, love and jealousy seem revolting or absurd, sexuality repulsive. . . .*

Where does this denial come from? Why the distorted perception of older people as asexual? Worst of all, why have *we* accepted another of the myths and stereotypes that cast us in the roles of the unimportant, the unfeeling, the insignificant? The reasons are complex, but if we examine them one by one, they become a fascinating study in how the absurd can become accepted as gospel.

Can you, even now, picture your parents having intercourse? If there is one generational truism that overlaps the era in which we were born, it is the inability of almost any young person to imagine his or her parent, or anyone else over 45, making love. It has not changed, even today, and not too long ago a young woman I know asked her mother, with a tinge of annoyance, "Why do you and daddy close the door when you go in your bedroom? What do you do in there?" Her mother drew herself up to her full five feet, one inch and responded, "The same thing that you and your boyfriend do when *you* close *your* door!"

It is as incomprehensible for that contemporary young woman to think of *her* parents making love as it was for us—and for our grandparents when they were young men and women. We were conceived through some act of sterile acrobatics, perhaps, and then it stopped. The interesting thing is that, until recently, no one even bothered to *ask* us if we continued our sexual interests after the birth of the children. As we got older, it became even more unusual for anyone to care. Dr. Alex Comfort observes that the sex surveys did not even include older people. The reason was that "everyone *knew* they had none, and they were assumed to have none, because nobody asked."

The times have certainly changed in terms of sexual attitudes, but many perceptions have remained exactly where they were 50 years ago. Recalling that *we* could not envision our parents or grandparents having intercourse, how interesting it is to note that our children are also unable to close that same emotional gap. And they are supposed to be liberated. We were retarded by comparison. Or were we?

At 17, I—like millions of my male contemporaries—was in a constant state of anticipatory tumescence. Little did I know that the girls of our generation were also sexual beings. The categories of girls were, of course, designated by our parents: good girls, fast girls, and bad girls. Since all the girls in our neighborhood were good girls, the perpetual ache in the loins was never to be sated by them. However, always the optimists, each of us carried a rolled-up condom in the small pocket of his wallet, where a permanent ridge formed and the protection lay there "just in case" we should get lucky and find one of those fast girls from another borough. The rubber lay there so long, in fact, that should we ever have had need for it, it probably would have disintegrated into a little puff of dust as we took it out of its hiding place! Nevertheless, the youths of our day retained their optimism.

William Styron in his book *Sophie's Choice* writes of a typical situation in those more naive days when his hero meets a girl from Brooklyn and, each time they are together, the sexual tension builds, only to have her pull back from the act of intercourse at the very last moment. It was true. It was, unfortunately—hilariously—devastatingly true. If we young men were lucky enough to meet a moderately "fast" girl, the ceremony of sexual petting took place through an array of medieval armor: brassiere fasteners and hooks, snaps, buttons, zippers, garters, and girdles. And if we were fortunate enough to finally make our way to the bare flesh that lay between girdle and stocking top, a firm hand usually reached out to stop us and a voice came from the darkness in a combination of worldliness and naiveté: "*What are you doing*?!" Somehow I could never figure out just why she didn't know what I was doing!

I never met one of those bad girls. If I wanted to change the contraceptive in my wallet just in case I did, I was always unlucky enough to find, upon walking into the drugstore, a woman clerk behind the counter. Muttering something about needing some toothpaste, I would purchase what I really did not need and shuffle out of the store, knowing that the protection that lay in my back pocket "just in case" would have to do for another year or two. It did have one side benefit: I never ran out of toothpaste.

Of course, the times have changed, and in many ways for the better. My corner druggist keeps his display of contraceptives right out on the counter. They are advertised in magazines. "Trojan: for Feeling in Love," and what a choice there is today! Trojan-enz, Trojan Ribbed, Trojan Plus, Ramses Intercept, Conceptrol Shields, Conceptrol Supreme, Fourex Natural Skins, Cavalier, and, with fanfare, "Stud 100: World-Famous Delay Spray for Men." All this and the Pill, the diaphragm, and the I.U.D.!

Have we, then, missed all this sexual liberation? We were born too soon to enjoy being able to shop for our contraceptives openly and without the furtive forays into the drugstore that had the same clandestine feeling as making a cocaine deal today. But, were there not many other things that more than adequately took the place of the sexual freedom and the "cold sex" that we read about now? Can we discard or minimize our feelings about commitment and caring, and was it so bad to "fall in love" so often? Were we wrong to demand that our displays of affection be made in private? We were, of course, different from the younger generations today, but so were *our* parents different from *us*.

As I walked along the beach last summer, while bathers dodged the strong waves of the Atlantic, a young couple lay near the dune line, their lower torsos barely covered with a jacket. Oblivious to the passersby, they were obviously having their own personal intercourse, the rhythms rising in telltale tension, her legs jumping like a rag doll's as he made love to her from behind. As I passed them I laughed, but not because of what they were doing. I remembered reading a lecture that Margaret Mead had delivered to a class of college women. "There's nothing that you do that we didn't do," she said, "only we didn't do it in front of the dean!"

But it does not stop. It does not, by any means, stop. The erotic relationships and sexual coupling may change, but there is no reason that it should terminate at some particular age. Our children and grandchildren may express the thought that we are finished with sex, but the obscenity occurs when we begin to believe them and we perpetuate the same myths. Over and over again, in the contemporary surveys that have been conducted among middle-aged and elderly people, the theory is reinforced by our own contemporaries, but when asked if *they* like sex, the retort is, generally, "Yes, but I'm an exception."

There are about 60 million "exceptions" in the country today, and it is becoming more evident to everyone that continuing sexual desire in middle and old age is not scandalous; that erotic relationships need not be kept clandestine; that this remarkable, earthy pleasure continues through our 50s, 60s, 70s, and well into our 80s. The perpetual tumescence in the male may be gone, but other changes take its place. In the words of Dr. Ruby Benjamin, a sex therapist with both a practical view of sex and a marvelous sense of humor, "Sexuality is more than the genital organs, the reproductive system, and the act of intercourse. It includes one's concept, partner choice, and patterns of interpersonal communication. The sex act is only one connection with sexuality. Aging can make the older person view sex as intimate communication in its best sense: tenderness, companionship, touching, caressing, the feelings of being needed and wanted, and the ability to give pleasure to another person and to receive it in return. All these are expressions of sexuality. The sensuous part of sexuality is as important, if not more important, than the sex act itself as we grow older."

All of this was borne out in still another study by Andrew Barclay, a psychologist, who reported in the journal *Medical Aspects of Human Sexuality* that even the sexual fantasies change with age. These fantasies, much like the sex drive, do not disappear, but their focus seems to dwell on a *wider variety* of sexual pleasures. He puts it beautifully when he writes, "It [the sex drive] may be thought of as a river which is narrow at its source, rushing noisily through rapids, but spreading out, slowing down, and meandering more as it approaches an outlet. We tend to find more things pleasurable as we age; we become less dependent upon sexual intercourse or genital contact as the sole expression of our sexuality."

The body changes, of course. Orgasm may take longer to achieve and may, in fact, occur only once in several acts of intercourse. In men, the erection may also take longer when compared to that of the young studs mentioned earlier, and it will certainly take more time between acts of intercourse for the erection to appear again. In women, the capacity for orgasm may also be slowed, though not terminated, by the aging process. The vagina may thin out and be less lubricated and elastic. But, as Dr. Benjamin says, "*all* physical responses are slowed as we age."

The most important thing to remember, however, is that, if there is a diminution of male sexual prowess and female responsiveness in the process of aging, it is usually due more to psychological rather than to biological reasons—boredom or preoccupation with the problems of family, the job, the financial situation; severe fatigue, or concerns about health, such as a recent heart attack.

The medical profession, as usual, has done little to counter the "bad press" that sex for the aging has received in our society. In direct contrast with many medical reports, a study by the National Institute on Aging showed that healthy older men maintain their production of sex hormones at levels found in younger men. In a further investigation, their scientists found that older men continue to ejaculate the same number of sperm as their young counterparts, though the proportion of immature sperm increases with age. Statisticians can, of course, point to the more than 20,000 men who become fathers after the age of 50.

But physicians, to no one's surprise, are as ill-informed and as subject to the myths of sex and aging as the general public. Dr. Benjamin says, "Some physicians and other health professionals, through sheer ignorance, can pass along destructive attitudes when they become aware of sex problems of older people. Some men and women look to their doctors for permission to express their sexuality for recreational purposes but, in fact, get the doctor's own personal, puritanical answers. In one study, 39 percent of the physicians questioned said that any woman over 50 should not *have* unfulfilled sexual needs. One would hardly expect an older woman to express her sexual desires and needs to one of *them!*"

Possibly we are throwing off the yoke, however burdened we have been with society's (and our own) view of ourselves as nonsexual hermits after the age of 50. Much of the psychological impotence in men is caused by the self-destructive view that it is inevitable that it will happen—and so it does.

For women, the self-image perpetuated by our youth culture can cause anxiety in those who feel that physical beauty is a fundamental requirement for sexual gratification. As Dr. Benjamin says, "I wonder when those cute little freckles of youth become those ugly age spots of the older woman. ... Older women—each of us—need to begin to command respect and admiration—not in spite of being older but because of it. Sexual image and self-image are at stake. We need to develop our own standards, not to compete with younger women."

About ten years ago it all began to surface, slowly at first but in an ever-increasing flow of articles, research studies, and news reports. Somehow, with wide-eyed wonder, the reporters, many of them young, began to write of retirement communities in Florida and Arizona and California where older people were discovered holding hands, dancing together, dating, kissing in public, and even becoming engaged and getting married again.

For those who did not want to marry, sometimes because the Social Security benefits would be reduced, there were "nonmarriages of convenience," very much like those of their children and grand-children. And instead of the stories being published as "exceptions," the flow began to increase and they are a remarkable object lesson both to our children and to those of us who think that "acting our age" is equated with giving up the pleasures of sex, whatever its form. A woman whom I interviewed told me that she had never enjoyed sex until she married for the second time. She was married for the second time at the age of 70!

More than 225,000 readers responded when "Dear Abby" asked in her column whether women over 50 enjoyed sex. Over 50 percent were enthusiastic in answering yes!

My uncle Jack remarried for the second time at the age of 89, his bride a mere snip of a lass at 82. Luckily the wedding was conducted in a cathedral in deference to the faith of the bride, and the church, not to be put off by stereotypes and myths, had my uncle sign a paper agreeing that the children would be brought up in the Catholic faith!

It is even happening in the hallowed halls of the nursing homes and the retirement residences, where society once refused to believe that older people have any feelings at all. On a visit to one such home I was invited to luncheon by the staff psychologist. One by one, the elderly came down to their midday meal. A 75-year-old woman in a wheelchair was pointed out to me and the man who pushed it toward the dining room was identified as her lover. He put her to bed every night, helped her to dress and undress, and spent his leisure hours talking to her and holding her hand. Years ago they both would have been expelled, for everyone knew that at 75 it was impossible to have a lover. But, today, there is the glimmer of a gradually changing attitude on the part of the patients and the administrators, both of whom no longer deny the need to touch, to hold, and to have sex if they want to. I can only hope that it becomes more universally true as administrative executives continue to become more enlightened. Unfortunately, the attitudes I have described are not yet universally accepted.

If all this is taking place at the age of 70 and older, why are we denying our sexuality in our 40s and 50s and 60s? It took me many years to discover and to admit to myself that my own mother was a sexual person, though she played the role of the '20s flapper right to her death and never would admit publicly what I am about to relate.

She traveled to Tulsa to visit my brother and his family and on the plane met a young woman doctor who was flying to meet her "special person." When my mother telephoned from Oklahoma, she said in her sotto voce tones, reserved for matters of personal and private import, "I was dying to ask her where she was going to stay when she got there." I told her that the young woman would probably stay with her boyfriend. "Not her," retorted my mother, "she was a *good* girl!" (There we go again—a *good* girl.) What my mother never admitted, however, was the fact that *she* had lived with my stepfather for *nine years* before they finally got married!

So sex lives! Dr. Benjamin even reports that there is evidence that sexual activity serves as therapy for arthritis sufferers "by increasing the adrenal-gland output of cortisone, thus alleviating the symptoms." However, she laughingly adds that she does not therefore advocate that, if you are suffering from arthritis, you grab the first partner you see and have sex for "medicinal purposes."

You might just think about one thing when it comes down to the image of ourselves as middle-aged people, our sexuality, and the fact that we are a generation that is finding new opportunities in all the areas of our lives. If you should weaken and cast a wistful, slightly envious eye at the younger generations and their open sexuality, lack of commitment, and the so-called "freedom" of their life styles, keep in mind that it has also brought a thousand other dissatisfactions into being. As they probe their own myths and stereotypes, trying to live up to what society thinks they are, it becomes more and more evident that the trade-offs are not as glorious as they would like us to believe. What they seem to have gained in physical freedom, they are beginning to feel they have lost in emotional depth.

Like us, they are also in constant state of change, of discovery, and of deep, sometimes very disturbed, personal soul-searching. Though they think of us as asexual, they are drawing back, more and more frequently, from contacts that have no depth and from relationships that involve no commitment. It was with a bit of wry chagrin and a smile of sympathy that I read a review of a new book written *for the young* by Dr. Gabrielle Brown. Finally, it was time to take a good hard look at this new era of sexual freedom. The book was titled *The New Celibacy*.

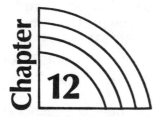

# In the Image of God

> *Joy, temperance, and repose*
> *Slam the door in the doctor's nose.*
> *Oliver Wendell Holmes*

I have always been amazed at the speed at which humor travels, and just as astonished at the endurance of some jokes, first told to me as a teen-ager and then recounted some 40 years later by the child of a friend, who then tells it as new-found gospel. If the humor has in it a basic truth or an element of hostility, it seems to spread even faster. Societies have been known to go on because of their sense of humor, their stories frequently hiding the deep conflicts of their political, economic, or social lives.

There is a long line in front of the Pearly Gates, as St. Peter checks the credentials of all who are to enter Heaven. The wait seems interminable, but since time is no longer of the essence, it doesn't seem to matter, until those assembled see a man in a white jacket, a stethoscope around his neck, walk briskly around the waiting crowd, past St. Peter and through the gates. An angry murmur arises, mutterings of "Who does he think he is?" St. Peter holds up his hand to calm them, saying, "Oh, that's God. He thinks he's a doctor!"

Not too long after hearing that joke for the fourth time, I was on a crowded airplane from Los Angeles to New York. The movie, which I half-watched and whose name I have since forgotten, starred Frank Sinatra and Faye Dunaway. Somewhere in the middle of the picture, poor Faye Dunaway is lying on her deathbed. Sinatra, unhappy with the treatment she is receiving, grabs her doctor by the lapels and angrily hurls him against the wall. The reaction in the plane was astounding. Three hundred people applauded and shrieked approval! The only ones who did not join in were those not watching the movie—unless they might have been doctors and their families.

What has happened to our gods? What, indeed, has happened to the benign, understanding, omniscient, omnipotent doctor of medicine? Was the doctor, in fact, *ever* a figure to be idolized? Or is it possible that *we* are as guilty of stereotyping *him* (or her), as he is of passing us off as "getting older, so what can you expect?" Have *we* perpetuated the myths about the doctor and did the doctor, in turn, begin believing all that gratifying public relations material he kept reading about himself? The folk hero. The steady-handed, sharp-eyed surgeon. The kindly *Saturday Evening Post* family physician. Commands given in the knowing tones of a U-boat captain. Follow the orders and you will live happily ever after. The image of the doctor as a god has, rightfully, become tarnished.

For those of us in our middle lives, medicine and the attitudes of our physicians play an even more important role in our well-being than they ever have before. It is quite true that chronic diseases increase as we age, though the incidence of acute conditions actually drops. Nutrition becomes more important to us—or at least it should. We—and our doctors—tend to turn more frequently to drugs as a panacea. Surgery soars at an alarming rate, most of it unnecessary, it seems. The prevailing attitude of the medical profession is that nothing can be done to cure many of our miseries because we are aging. Add to that all the other failings of specialists trained only to treat one or two specific diseases rather than try to prevent them in the first place. Finally, consider the appalling rigidity of the American Medical Association toward anything new and innovative. Soon it becomes clear that the doctor can actually be a threat to us as we age—that is, unless we know the nature of our problems and some of the solutions that have been discovered, and unless we take an active role in our health care.

So it is high time that we take a harder look at our beloved family doctors and their surgical friends. It is time to return to an important member of the "middle-age hit list."

# More Myths, More Stereotypes

A medical publication, *Pediatric News* published an article some time ago commenting on the fact that "physicians behave differently toward a patient depending upon the patient's race, sex, age, and personal appearance." The article went on to suggest that doctors look more carefully at their attitudes to make certain that *everyone* receives "courteous and empathetic care."

But doctors are, after all, people, so why should we expect them to feel any different when the prejudice toward the aging of our society is found on every level, even among *ourselves*? Unfortunately, the field of medicine is not insulated in some magical way from the rest of our imperfect world, so it is not surprising that the doctor also develops a demeaning, superficial, false, and stereotypical view of aging.

If *we* are subjected to a constant barrage of media stereotypes about aging, so is the physician, even in his own medical journals. One survey analyzed 151 drug advertisements that appeared in the journal *Geriatrics* over a 20-year period. Though as time passed the number of women in the ads increased and a more positive view of elderly persons began to emerge, a large number of the ads portrayed the older adult as either sad, ill, incompetent, or withdrawn. In addition, over 30 percent of the headlines in the ads showing the elderly were negative.

Add to this the fact that the medical schools barely touch upon geriatric medicine, and you begin to understand the diagnosis, "Well, you're getting older, what can you expect?" or the all-encompassing catchword explanation, "senescence."

The myths of aging are so pervasive that we begin to believe—and our doctors share the view—that as we grow older *all of us* complain about our health, worry excessively about our physical condition, and visit the doctor's office with a severe case of hypochondria at the slightest sign of malaise. Of course, there are some who do just that, but the National Institute on Aging issued a report in 1980 that said, in part, "While it is true that certain health problems do increase with age, there is no evidence that health complaints are disproportionate among older people. . . . Specifically, older people report more problems with the sensory, cardiovascular, and genito-urinary systems. This is not surprising, since these systems are known to be more susceptible to disease and disability with increasing age." The report concluded that the proportion of people who might be considered hypochondriacal is no higher among the middle-aged and aged than it is among the young!

We have been so conditioned by society that we take it for granted that we will have aches and pains as we reach middle age. And so do our doctors. We accept the myth that we will deteriorate rapidly after the age of 50 and the mind will disintegrate into irreversible senility, to live in a shadow world of depression and confusion. And our doctors, too many of them, believe that too. It is true that our *speed* of response declines as we age, but it has been proven time and time again that most older people maintain a normal level of vigorous mental capacity right up to their deaths at 85 or 90. Alex Comfort points out that less than *1 percent* of all people become senile—a smaller percentage than that of young people who go insane!

I have heard too many young people tell me that their grandparents were aging and that it was time to put them in a nursing home. They are being conditioned along with the rest of us, accepting this as a link in an inevitable chain of events in spite of the fact that it is yet another myth. Only 4 to 5 percent of the elderly are in nursing homes! Another 5 percent are homebound because of illness. As a matter of fact, only 15 percent of the population over the age of 65 is in any need of special health or social services. That leaves *85 percent* who are still active in their homes and communities.

One of the most appalling responses of the medical profession is to label, automatically, the symptoms of confusion, depression, memory loss, or deteriorating judgment as "senility" or "senescence," just because the patient is getting older. These signs may very well be caused by dozens of other *treatable* diseases, by improper nutrition, *or by the drugs being prescribed by one's physician*, as we shall see later on. But if you should question your doctor about a diagnosis, prognosis, or treatment, the response frequently resembles that given a child who asks a precocious question—a mixture of amusement and disdain. If so, it may be time to find a new family doctor!

# Intervention—Not Prevention

There is a temptation to offer a small apology when modern medicine is taken to task. I was brought up in the era of reverence toward the family doctor, and my own physician today, Dr. Bob Levin, is a classic and shining exception to everything negative that I feel and that I write about on this subject. In dealing with the average doctor, each criticism I make is countered with a request for the name of the medical school that I attended. After all, if I am not an M.D., how can I even begin to know how to phrase my questions, much less criticize Hippocrates and his fellow travelers?

My wife once asked our former family physician just what the side effects would be for a drug that he had prescribed for my aging mother-in-law. His answer was, "It's better you shouldn't know!"

I think it is time for modern medicine to agree that we have a right to know, a right to be involved in monitoring our own health and well-being. Doctors are aware that more and more of us are questioning, probing, and exploring new approaches. We are terribly disturbed at the reaction we get from the stubborn kingdom that derives so much of its power from our own trust, so often misplaced. Too many of us have "horror" stories about medical care. It is no wonder that we have begun to question more deeply, to ask for answers long denied us, to demand that we be *heard*.

I watched an early-morning television program in Los Angeles several months ago, fascinated by an interview with Dr. Robert S. Mendelsohn, author of *Confessions of a Medical Heretic* (Contemporary Books, Chicago, 1979) and a more recent work, *Male Practice: How Doctors Manipulate Women* (Contemporary Books, Chicago, 1981). Impressed by the man and his thinking, I immediately read the latter book and then telephoned him at his office in Illinois. If he felt so strongly about the mistreatment of women by gynecologists, obstetricians, and general practitioners, was there a parallel in medicine for the aging? After all, he mentioned that almost 700,000 hysterectomies were performed in the United States in 1979 and that *not more than one in five could even be considered clinically necessary!* It seemed to be a classic case involving more than half of our generation: being a woman and aging at the same time.

> *I don't think there's any question about the fact that what I've written about women and gynecology is also a fact about medicine for the aging. . . . Discrimination against the aged in medicine—it's just all over the place. You can make the case against medicine and you can make the same case against medical education, since students take*

*geriatric medicine only as an elective. They learn nothing
about older folks!*

Yet these same graduates treat older patients as a part of their
internship and residency, and eventually in their private practice? "Yes,"
he answered, "It pays their office rent!"

There are about 125 major medical schools in the country today,
yet only about 25 to 30 of them are seriously committed to any study
of aging and geriatric medicine. Dr. Robert N. Butler, writing in a report
for *Geriatrics* (National Institute on Aging), asserted, "The needs of
older people have been much neglected in the training of health professionals, in the structuring and financing of medical services, and in the
support of biomedical and behavioral research. Medical school curricula
generally do not reflect the incidence and character of the multiple
disorders of old age. Medicare is designed as if its beneficiaries were
young. . . ."

Some medical schools are becoming aware of the problem, though
I am not quite certain that the results are what they had expected them
to be. The Medical College of Pennsylvania has instituted a program
designed to help its young medical students become aware of the problems of the aging patients they will one day treat. With simulated han-
dicaps such as blindness, failing hearing, crippling from arthritis, the
students are required to accomplish simple tasks such as preparing
dinner or taking a book off a library shelf. I would expect these young
people to come out of the exercise thoroughly empathetic with the aging
population. Too often, the opposite happens. The *New York Times* reported this comment from one medical student, her ears plugged with
cotton, her hands tightly bound in rubber gloves to limit mobility and
dexterity, trying to use the telephone and get a correct number from
the information operator: *"It sure makes you want to stay young!"*
(Italics mine.)

While such specialties as nuclear medicine, pediatric roentgen-
ology, and neonatology take precedence in medical schools today, "the
long-standing deficiencies in geriatric teaching represent the uncon-
scious negative attitudes toward the elderly that permeate our society,"
Dr. Butler says. In the course of a medical education, the student will
learn about a *quarter-million* separate pieces of information, very few
of them relating to aging.

There are probably many subconscious factors that add to the
inadequacy of our medical treatment as we grow older. The aging pa-

tient is no longer as aesthetically appealing as the younger one, and one result is that many examinations, as well as the communication of "caring," are performed less diligently if at all. Overmedication and hasty, unnecessary surgical intervention follow these encounters all too often. At a dinner party one evening I heard a young gynecologist remark that he was "turned on" when he examined his younger female patients. Does that shock you? We have already admitted that some of our gods are really people.

Incidentally, there is an immediate reaction when someone mentions a male gynecologist who is less than adequate, too rough, or unsympathetic. "Go to a woman doctor," is the response. Sometimes it works, but remember that most of the women practicing medicine have been trained by *men*. The men run the medical schools and they run the profession. Don't be surprised if the female doctor reflects exactly the same predispositions and prejudices as her male colleagues.

In the field of surgery, the victims are of all ages, but unfortunately the threat increases as we grow older. It has been estimated that only 20 percent of all operations performed today are essential—serious trauma or cancer surgery, for example, and other procedures required to save or to extend a patient's life. The rest are questionable or unneeded.

Where the finances are in direct relationship to the number of operations performed, the statistics rise in skyscraper leaps. Hospitals need to fill beds in order to survive inflationary costs. In addition, there are about 30 percent too many surgeons in a country already rich with medical practitioners, and all of them are trying to make a living. Dr. Peter Bourne, ex-President Carter's special assistant for health issues, put it more succinctly: "If one has to be really blunt about it, there's an economic incentive—the more surgery you do, the more money you get."

The expanding health insurance plans have also made surgery more available and more affordable. And so, by no real coincidence, the number of elective operations performed in the United States has soared— and most of the patients could have done better without them. During the 1970s, the number of operations rose 23 percent while the population increased only by 11 percent. Caesarean sections almost doubled, cataract extractions increased by over 40 percent, and prostatectomies rose by about the same figure. Not to our credit, the United States now has the highest hysterectomy rate in the world. It is more than twice that of Great Britain and four times the rate of Sweden! With all this, of course, the death rate from surgery has also soared.

The doctors, of course, have an answer. Dr. Mendelsohn writes, "When doctors are charged with overmedicating their patients, the typical response is, 'the patient wanted it.' This 'blame the victim' strategy is one that doctors employ to cover most of their sins, whether the transgression lies in pushing drugs or performing hysterectomies and Caesarean sections that their patients shouldn't have and don't need."

Somehow I cannot accept the premise that "we ask for it." The surgeons state that we put the pressure on them to perform surgery, that they are really doing it for us. A British surgeon, interviewed by a newspaper reporter, recounted the classic medical joke about the compliant patient. The doctor says, "Mrs. Smith, we're scheduling you for a decapitation next Wednesday," and Mrs. Smith answers, "Fine."

The only defense I can accept on the part of doctors practicing today is the soaring malpractice insurance premiums due to a plague of insurance cases leveled against the profession, with the concomitant multi-million dollar awards. As a result, many doctors have begun to practice "defensive" medicine, ordering many tests and writing many prescriptions with the thought that ignoring any avenue of diagnosis or medication might well result in a lawsuit. I accept that and I acknowledge the problem. All I ask is that, in return, the medical profession try to understand how *we* feel during that visit to the doctor.

Frightened, vulnerable, alone, trusting, looking for an answer from someone we believe is an idol (and who believes it half the time himself), potentially ill or suffering from what we've just been told is a possibly fatal illness if we don't do something about it right away— that instant!—what does the surgeon expect us to say; how does he expect us to react?

There are things we *must* learn to do. Dr. Mendelsohn advises, "Don't reinforce your doctor's feelings of omnipotence by allowing or encouraging him to patronize and intimidate you. Be on your guard, and make him explain and defend every diagnosis he makes, every drug he prescribes, every operation he recommends. Don't be in awe of him. Compel him to accept you as an equal, because you deserve his respect at least as much as he merits yours!"

And if surgery is recommended? Don't be afraid to get a second opinion. If necessary, Dr. Mendelsohn urges that you get on a plane and fly to some other city where the doctor has no connection with your own surgeon. Tell him, by the way, that, whatever his diagnosis, *he* will not be retained to perform the operation. If you're still in doubt, get a *third* opinion, and don't be rushed into anything.

A few days ago I found an epitaph written by Matthew Prior at the beginning of the 18th century. As the surgery boom increases, it might be well noted today: "Cured yesterday of my disease, I died last night of my physician."

# Hospitals Can Be Hazardous to Your Health

A few years ago Lois Gould wrote a novel called *Such Good Friends*, in which the husband of the heroine goes into the hospital for the removal of a wart, a simple operation. While undergoing surgery he dies of "complications." There is, of course, a word to describe this contingency that seems to be *increasing* rather than diminishing over these last few decades. It is a marvelously fluid word, one that rolls easily off the tongue and makes us sound well-read and knowledgeable. It is "iatrogenesis," and it is such a superb word that I wish it did not describe so awful a situation—the risks of illness and medical complications that occur during a medical procedure for something entirely different. The situation described by Lois Gould would be just such an iatrogenic event. And the hospital, always a leader in "medibabble," would term an iatrogenic infection as "nosocomial" (hospital-related), another likely candidate for the chapter on future-talk.

Dr. Mendelsohn writes, "Hospitals *look* awesomely antiseptic. They are actually so germ-laden that 5 percent of all hospital patients contract infections that they didn't have when they arrived. As a result, they are stuck there for an average of seven extra days."

In one hospital, a study showed that 36 out of 2,500 patients admitted for surgery suffered mild to severe complications because of mistakes by physicians! And of those 36, 20 died, with 11 of the deaths directly linked to doctor error. Of the 16 who survived, 5 had serious physical impairment that could have been avoided. A story in the *Wall Street Journal* concluded that "most of the complications were due to poor judgment by the surgeon. Such problems included reaching the wrong diagnosis, delaying needed surgery, performing unnecessary or overextensive surgical procedures, or ignoring trouble signs because of overconfidence or misplaced optimism."

For those of us who are entering our middle years and are soon to be numbered among the elder segment of our population, the hazards of hospitalization should not be underestimated. Given the combination of an increasing number of chronic ailments and the penchant of doctors and surgeons to recommend some sort of drastic remedy, from drugs to major surgery, the risks of a hospital stay, no matter what its duration, are not trivial.

The National Institute on Aging reported on a study by the Boston University School of Medicine in which over *one-third* or 290 patients out of 815 studied suffered medical complications as a result of being hospitalized. Of these 76 had more than one major complication. Iatrogenesis contributed to the deaths of 15 of the victims. Drugs accounted for 208 iatrogenic events, diagnostic heart procedures for 45, and falls for 35. "Another problem," the report goes on, "was that medical records . . . frequently failed to comment upon or even note apparently significant iatrogenic events."

Note, if you will, the largest number in the foregoing list. Now I'd like you to meet a business partner of the medical profession—the pharmaceutical concerns

# Our Aging Junkies

Voltaire wrote, "Physicians have been pouring drugs about which they know little for diseases about which they know less into beings about whom they know nothing." Since Americans over the age of 50 take about 25 percent of all drugs prescribed by doctors (and many that are not), this is still another area that concerns us, especially since chronic illness is an occasional companion of a longer life span.

We have reached a point where both we and our doctors expect that there is "a pill for every ill." If we happen to suffer from more than one illness, real or hypochondriacal, we begin to mix our pills—sometimes prescribed by more than one doctor, each unaware of the other's prescription!

"What is the response going to be when you take two drugs that conflict—or two drugs in combination with a nutritional item . . . is it compatible with orange juice, for example, or liquor?" I was visiting St. Barnabas Hospital in the Bronx, where I had produced two films some years ago, one of them on chronic disease and aging. Janet Beard, who heads the Braker Home, sat at lunch with me and Dr. Manny Riklan. "I'm not too sure that the doctors know the response. I'm not too sure they take the time to read the literature—they get it from one side only, from the pharmaceutical side, and not from the pharmacological side."

For the doctor, there is a constant stream of new drugs that enter the market as panaceas for high blood pressure, diabetes, glaucoma, arthritis, heart attacks, cancer, digestive disturbances, and all the other diseases that can strike us as we age. At one time a stroke could dispatch us with relative speed; today there are drugs that can keep us active and alive for 20 years or more.

Much of the doctor's knowledge comes from the salespeople who work for the pharmaceutical concerns, and very few doctors have time to read the literature that accompanies the samples flowing into every physician's office every day of the year. A veritable cornucopia of wonder drugs! Or are they?

We *expect* the doctor to give us a prescription when we leave his office. He is, in fact, taught in medical school to give us something to take with us. A little token in Latin makes it all worthwhile. Too often the prescription is for a drug about which he knows little, though he prescribes it with great confidence, and he gives us no information about what the side effects may be.

I mentioned earlier that my wife had been told by a doctor to give her ailing and aging mother Thorazine and he, in his wisdom, answered her question about side effects with, "It's better you shouldn't know." She went immediately to the pharmacist and looked in his reference book. Much to her horror, the side effects were potentially worse than the condition for which they were prescribed! Not only that: since most drugs today are tested on young and middle-aged people, the dosage for an elderly, frail, sickly woman of 85 pounds seemed terribly high. She cut the dosage herself and I quite forgot about Thorazine until I found an incredible story in Dr. Mendelsohn's book, a classic "chicken and egg" tale.

Thorazine is prescribed for psychic disorders: agitation, excessive anxiety, and tension. However, some of its side effects are symptoms resembling those of Parkinson's disease. When a side effect appears, the doctors then prescribe Artane, which has, in turn, its own side effects:

*Dizziness, nausea, psychotic manifestations, delusions, hallucinations, mental confusion, agitation, and disturbed behavior.*

Naturally, when *these* side effects are reported to the family physician, he immediately recommends another drug to counteract them: Thorazine!

Again we are vulnerable, for even the doctor knows too little about drug incompatibilities and side effects, and the pharmaceutical companies are in a profit-motive industry. The more they sell, the more they make. Of course, the drugs have all been tested and approved by the Food and Drug Administration. And of course, the drug companies spend millions of dollars on research and on the advertising and promotion that gets their product into the hands of physicians too busy to study its effects. Thalidomide was tested and researched. DES (diethylstilbestrol) has surfaced as the villain in vaginal cancer in the daughters of women in our generation who were given the drug during pregnancy. Bendectin, a supposedly well-researched and tested drug for morning sickness, is now being blamed for many of the same birth defects that were caused by thalidomide.

As we age, the horror stories multiply. Cases of drug misuse and misinformation are so common in our aging population that they seem to be the rule rather than the exception. There are stories of senior citizens sampling one another's pills. Drug toxicity emergencies rise as the population ages. Consumers aged 50 and over are the biggest market for over-the-counter drugs. We buy 60 percent of all arthritic and rheumatic pain relievers, 45 percent of all laxatives, and 25 percent of all nonprescription drugs, a market of $1.3 billion! Yet there are many over-the-counter drugs that have dramatic and sometimes damaging side effects when taken either alone or in combination with other prescription drugs.

For example, in the book *Nonprescription Drugs* by the editors of *Consumer Guide* (Beekman House, New York, 1979), even a quick perusal is enough to make us sit up and take notice. I stood in the aisle of my local bookshop and opened the book to Chlor-Trimeton, a decongestant and cold allergy remedy sold over-the-counter and manufactured by the Schering Corporation. In addition to the warnings and contraindications for persons with peptic ulcers, glaucoma, heart and kidney disease, and other ailments, the potential side effects include: increased blood pressure, nervousness, anxiety, tension, insomnia, tremor, dizziness, headache, sweating, nausea, vomiting, loss of appetite, palpitations, chest pain, difficult or painful urination, blurred vision, confusion, constipation, and rash. All these—and the drug is in the nonprescription category! It makes me wonder just what medical time bombs are ticking away in the medications that are "just what the doctor ordered."

A classic and tragic case in point was published in the newspapers not long ago in the midst of a severe summer heat spell. Three psychiatric patients in state hospitals died when the temperature soared over 95 degrees and the humidity rose to extreme levels. The patients were in wards that had no air conditioning and only small slits in the windows. They were all on antipsychotic drugs. The side effects of the drugs? They lower the ability of the patient to withstand severe heat!

"Another thing with aging people," Janet Beard says, "if you look in their medicine cabinets, they have outdated drugs, some from one doctor and some from another. Doctor A doesn't know what Doctor B gave them. We call them 'medical shoppers' and what we try to say to them is that you need *one* person to coordinate your health."

Each of the drugs in your medicine cabinet may be safe and each may be effective for the particular condition for which it was prescribed, but the "polypharmacy" that lies there can be dangerous if taken at the same time and if you are not completely familiar with potential side effects. In addition, many of the tranquilizers that are prescribed so readily today may well be habit-forming, and when you finally decide that you don't need the Miltown or Valium, the effects of withdrawal will make it almost impossible to give them up. Before you quickly condemn heroin and marijuana, it might be wise to look more carefully at those rows of neat bottles of "establishment" drugs that line your medicine cabinet.

What, then, can we do? The answer is at once simple and complex. We must learn to protect ourselves from the quick and easy prescribing of drugs by our doctors (abetted by the sales pitches of the pharmaceutical concerns) by acquiring as much knowledge as we can about what is being peddled to us. Don't expect your doctor to cooperate easily. If he is like most medical practitioners, even broaching a simple question is tantamount to heresy. Be firm and insist that he respond to your questions—if he won't, find another doctor.

🖋 Ask your physician what the side effects of the prescribed drug might be. Are there any warnings of reactions or interactions that you should know about?

🖋 Discuss with the doctor any other medications you are taking and for what conditions. Include over-the-counter medicines, laxatives, and vitamins.

🖋 Try to write down what the doctor tells you about what he/she prescribes. Most of us are so tense during a medical visit that we tend to forget the instructions, or we may think they'll be perfectly clear on the medicine bottle. Is the pill taken on an empty stomach, after breakfast, before bedtime? Should you avoid driving after taking the prescribed dose?

⧆ Is the doctor, in fact, giving you the smallest possible dose to attack the problem? I have never been able to understand why a 100-pound female may be given exactly the same dosage as a 200-pound male.

⧆ If you should develop side effects, report them to the doctor at once. And if your physician then tries to prescribe still another drug to eliminate the side effects, you had better question him even more rigorously!

There is one more point and it has to do with the economics of the drug world. The pharmaceutical companies would like you to use only their brand-name medications and they do what they can to encourage the doctors to prescribe Miltown, for example, rather than the generic meprobamate. Both are the same drug but brand-name drugs are expensive and, in many cases, a waste of your money. Certainly there may be a time when a particular drug is recommended because of patient sensitivity or the fine-tuning of a specific brand. But one survey in New York found that the vast majority of brand-name prescriptions were written for the commonest of painkillers, tranquilizers, antihistamines, diet drugs, and antibiotics. Each year patients in New York City alone were paying over $10 million too much for the privilege of using a brand name.

Publication of the report immediately brought a typical response from the president of the state medical society, in which he assailed the very idea of using generic drugs, claiming that brand names allowed the physician to use his "vital experiential techniques . . . and close monitoring of a patient's response" in prescribing a "drug with which he is completely familiar." I wish I could believe him, especially that last part, for all evidence seems to point to the contrary and it would be a good idea to ask your doctor what generic drug can replace the one he has prescribed—and then have a discussion with your neighborhood pharmacist.

Ideally, I wish we could all follow Sir William Osler's advice that a doctor's first duty is "to educate the masses not to take medicine." Failing that, just amend the statement made by our ex-family physician: "It's better you *should* know!"

# How to Shop for a Doctor

With it all, we need our physicians, even our surgeons. Not even the angriest of modern medicine's critics would suggest that we return to the practices of the past century, at least not in a technological sense. (There is no doubt that we would like to reinstitute house calls and empathy.) But so much energy has been devoted to the treatment of sickness rather than the maintenance of good health; the expansion of a complex and expensive hospital system rather than the advancement of nutrition and disease prevention; a dependence on our doctors rather than taking responsibility for ourselves, that both we and our physicians have become trapped in a spiral of impersonal and inflationary medical care.

In instances of acute illness, when we *must* see a physician, we are frequently left with an inadequate choice. As people who are in midlife, it is inconceivable that we should be without medical help when we actually need it. Yet many of us feel anger, hostility, and fear toward a profession we were taught to admire and to accept without question.

We shop for our automobiles with care and with exquisite attention to minute details of performance, appearance, and durability. Our refrigerators are purchased on the basis of thorough investigation by Consumer's Union and the references of neighbors and friends. If the accountant should make a serious error in our income tax returns, we would strongly consider changing accountants. And if our grocer treated us with the same lack of human concern shown by some of our doctors, we would certainly begin shopping around. Why, then, do we accept from the medical profession—when our health and our lives are at stake—what we would not tolerate from anyone else? Let us first of all take a good, hard, realistic view of our physicians, taking note of the saying that my wife likes to quote: "Remember, 50 percent of all doctors graduated in the lower half of their class!" Then let us shop for our doctors with the same care and attention to detail that we give to purchasing our new automobiles.

## I Want a Doctor Who Can Separate My Chronological Age from My Physical Condition. I am no more prone to aches and pains than I was 10 years or 20 years ago; I am no crazier, nor am I more senile, and neither are most of my peers. As a matter of fact, I probably was more crazy at 17 than I am now.

**I Want a Doctor Who Is Open to New Ideas.** Medicine is too quick to turn obdurate at the first suggestion of an idea that goes against its teaching or threatens its status. It took poor Dr. Ignaz Semmelweis a torturously long time to convince his colleagues that postpartum infection was caused by their not washing their hands before a delivery. The posture of medicine has not changed very much since then. I want my family physician to accept the holistic concept of medicine: that I am a whole person who is suffering from a disease. I resent anyone's referring to me in a hospital as "the gallbladder" or "the hernia," as so many physicians seem to do. If I discuss chiropractic with my doctor, I would like the courtesy of a hearing and a discussion of a drug-free, surgery-free alternative, rather than being dismissed with a sigh of resignation or the vituperative evaluation "Quack!"

I want the same response and openness of acceptance if I ask about acupuncture, biofeedback, the Feldenkrais method or the Jacobson technique, Rolfing, shiatsu, yoga, Gestalt, or homeopathy.

If there is a disfiguring or life-saving operation involved, then I certainly want my doctor to be open to new therapies, new techniques, new approaches. Certainly, if I were a woman of my age, I would want to know much more about the alternatives in treatment open to me if I were to find a small lump in my breast one morning. For years many surgeons have accepted the Halsted radical mastectomy as the only solution to breast cancer, though newer and more desirable techniques have evolved. I was present in a surgeon's office when he recommended immediate hospitalization and surgery to take care of a lump on the breast. When asked for the alternatives, or what would happen if nothing were done, he turned condescendingly, almost hostilely and asked, "Am I hearing you correctly?" The patient walked out, never to return. The surgery he was recommending, incidentally, turned out to be unnecessary.

There are times when it is not only the doctor who has a closed mind to new ideas, but the entire medical profession. Frankly, I worry about it. When I produced my Academy Award nomination film *To Live Again* (1963), I had the honor and the pleasure of working with the brilliant neurosurgeon, Dr. Irving Cooper at St. Barnabas Hospital in the Bronx, New York. A young man at the time, he had recently developed a remarkable operation that involved working deep within the brain for relief of the symptoms of parkinsonism. The technique, cryosurgery, required the insertion of a probe into the thalamus, then lowering the temperature in that area to below freezing to halt the incapacitating tremors or the rigidity of dystonia in patients who had appeared to be totally destroyed as human beings by the disease.

I watched him perform operation after operation, always in awe at the results—the tremors stopping as the patient lay awake on the table, fingers able to move, hands able to function. I fully expected the medical profession to rise in one loud cheer of acclaim, but it did not happen! Dr. Cooper, unfortunately, was "too young." Others who had attempted similar operations had failed, either through paralyzing their patients or by killing them altogether. Though he has operated successfully on over 6,000 patients, there are some doctors who, as late as 1980, still believe that he is a fraud, that he uses hypnosis, and possibly that he is a witch doctor, I imagine. Recently, he published a book, *The Vital Probe* (Norton, New York, 1981), a remarkable and sensitive history of his medical life. I recommend it to anyone who thinks that I am exaggerating when I condemn the world of medicine for being rigid, unyielding, and closed to new ideas.

## I Want My Questions Answered.

I don't want to be passed off with "Am I hearing you correctly?" or "It's better you shouldn't know." I don't want to be treated with a lack of respect and I don't want to be patronized. I demand integrity and I demand accountability in the answers my doctor gives. And I want *time* to discuss my questions and get the answers. I realize that "time is money," but my health is more important to me—and it should be to my physician.

## I Want a Doctor Who Is Conservative in His Treatment.

There is generally time to discuss, time to consider, time to decide if a major procedure is indicated, especially in the elective area of surgery. I want my doctor to be stingy with recommendations of surgery, drugs, or extensive testing. In a recent survey, nearly half the registered nurses across the country believed that between 30 and 50 percent of all operations and up to 50 percent of all hospital stays were unnecessary. I resent any diagnosis that might make me part of that statistic. We have a marvelous physician here at Fire Island in the summer, named Dr. Bob Furie, who is more to my liking. The doctor suggested to a friend of mine, who had been feeling unwell for a week or so, that he would be watching him, and in the meantime would treat him with "intensive neglect." The treatment worked, even though it is probably not taught in medical school.

**I Want a Doctor Who Values a Second Opinion.** It is not a sign that I lack confidence in my own family physician that I sometimes want the opinion of another doctor in a case more serious than the Asian flu. I would, in fact, appreciate *his* suggestion that I see another doctor to confirm or deny the diagnosis. As I advised earlier, if you do go for a second opinion, make sure you tell the surgeon or physician that *he* will not be the one who will treat you.

During a particularly difficult time in my own family's medical history, I read a remarkable book by Rose Kushner, *Why Me?* (Harcourt, Brace, Jovanovich, New York, 1975) an account of her own experience with breast cancer. Over a period of several weeks I spoke with her by telephone at her home in Maryland. Her support helped tremendously through that trying period. Along with a growing number of people in the medical profession, she strongly advocates that a woman undergo a two-stage approach to the breast biopsy, and that she never go into an operating room not knowing whether she will come out with only one breast intact.

It is just as important, she insists, that the patient obtain a second opinion, realizing that there is *time* to do it; she should not, must not, be rushed by the surgeon into a disfiguring and emotionally devastating operation. Her analogy, as strong and direct as she is, was delivered in a speech at a Women's Health Fair in Miami: "If you had a $50,000 Rolls Royce and it developed a knock, would you drive it into the nearest service station? Would you accept the corner mechanic's estimate of what was wrong—especially if he said it would cost $10,000 and he couldn't even guarantee it for six months? Of course not. You'd get another mechanic. And that's certainly what you should do for your body."

**I Want a Doctor Who Chooses Home over Hospital Where He Can.** If I am ill, I want to be surrounded by loved ones and pampered a bit and have homemade chicken soup when I need it. In most cases I am better off at home, while modern medicine chooses the hospital as the first and last resort. As a matter of fact, too many doctors choose the hospital as the final stop in a terminal illness when the patient would be much better off in his or her own home. It is an ongoing conflict between the philosophy of humanity and the pragmatics of medicine. The medical profession fights violently against a baby's being born at home and it is just as rigid in recommending that we also die in the isolation of a hospital room. It is changing slowly, but only through the pressures of patients and families.

### Above All, I Want a Doctor Who Believes in Prevention.
I want a doctor who likes me but doesn't really want to see me, because he and I both believe that a great part of the preventive role in medicine is *my* responsibility. Should I genuinely need him, I want him to be available to me, for I will only call when the necessity is real.

Doctors are becoming more aware and awareness may well be the first step on the road to change in attitudes. A research economist, speaking at a meeting of the American Society of Internal Medicine, commented that many patients are, indeed, questioning who is responsible for their state of health, and they are discovering that the duty is theirs rather than their physician's. He went on to say that increased attention to diet and exercise by patients would affect the livelihood of doctors, as fewer and fewer people would seek medical care. Somehow they will survive our independence!

*Pediatric News* carried an item in which a psychologist recommended that doctors give their patients a questionnaire at least once a year. "A patient questionnaire is an excellent practice management tool. It also is a superb patient relations tool; the request for their input sends out to patients a strong message: 'We care.' "

I certainly hope they do.

# An Apple a Day: Prevention—Not Intervention

During World War I my father was wounded three times, once quite seriously when gangrene began to infect his injured leg. One morning as he lay in a field hospital, a surgeon approached his bedside, handed him a piece of paper, and asked him to sign.

"What for?" my father asked. He was only 19 at the time.

"We have to amputate your leg to save your life," the doctor answered perfunctorily.

My father pushed the paper aside, turned away and said, "Not me. I was born with two legs and I'm going to die with two legs."

The gangrene disappeared and my father survived the war intact. For *60 years* afterward he never visited a physician. "I don't like doctors,

I don't trust doctors," he would say every time I tried to convince him that a current illness might well be looked at. And he was always right.

Just a few years ago my father hurt his wrist while at work and, after a few days of pain, I convinced him that it might well be a slight break, which it proved to be. Reluctantly he visited my family doctor with me and, as he took the medical history, the doctor asked, "When was the last time you visited a physician?" My father answered, "Nineteen-eighteen." The doctor looked up and smiled. "You're none the worse for it!"

The responsibility and many of the decisions that relate to our health and well-being arc actually up to us. We are finding that common sense approaches to health are far more effective than technology and sophisticated medical techniques. The American medical profession is self-laudatory in its public relations, yet an infant is safer being born in Denmark, Japan, Belgium, the Netherlands, Switzerland, Finland, or even Singapore than here in the United States. Fourteen other countries have better life expectancy statistics than the United States and, in spite of the self-acclaim of modern medicine, today's 45-year-old male can look forward to living only three to four years longer than his counterpart in 1900! And that was before the age of miracle drugs and the marvels of 20th-century surgery! (It is in the area of childhood disease that medicine has been most successful, thus allowing *more of us to live longer.*)

Doctors cannot give us our health habits. Weight control, regular exercise, good nutrition, not smoking, and avoiding excessive intake of alcohol are all part of *our* responsibility to ourselves, not the obligation of our doctors. In the past year the AMA suggested that we eliminate the routine annual physical examination. This was taken a step further by Dr. Mendelsohn when he wrote, "The door to the doctor's office ought to bear a surgeon general's warning that routine physical examinations are dangerous to your health. Many studies over the last decade or so have established that the annual physical examination is a waste of money and a waste of time."

Research groups around the world are beginning to discover that more and more of our diseases of aging either are caused by or can be cured by diet and nutrition. Osteoporosis, or brittleness of the bone, for example, is an important disease among older women and is generally associated with almost 200,000 hip fractures a year. New Zealand researchers have found that a low-calcium and high-salt diet may well lead to an increased risk of developing the disease, while the National

Institute on Aging issued a report indicating that a balanced diet with adequate levels of calcium and vitamins, sufficient exercise, and avoidance of cigarette smoking and heavy drinking, might help in *preventing* the onset of osteoporosis.

Small segments of the medical profession are also beginning to move into the area of *wellness* rather than sickness. The Gerontology Research Center of the National Institute on Aging is beginning to investigate such areas as adult nutrition, geriatric medicine, and the pharmacology of aging while attempting to promote mandatory courses in geriatric medicine in the medical schools, where it is now passed off as an elective subject.

Occasionally we also hear of an innovative and enlightened program that throws off the straitjacket of previous medical treatment and opens potentially new frontiers of preventive medicine. Mt. Sinai Hospital in New York has begun a new $4 million program devoted to improving the *quality* of life of the aging. St. Barnabas Hospital in the Bronx has instituted satellite health centers, in an outreach program brought right into the community itself. "The hospitals and the medical community have a role in teaching about smoking, about losing weight, about high blood pressure and how to check your own," Dr. Manny Riklan told me; "a health education program *before* you get sick."

Five such centers serve the community and in each of them a health educator teaches about hypertension, what foods to eat, what foods to avoid, exercise, and the treatment of diabetes and arthritis. "The programs are run just like a college," Dr. Riklan explained, "with the 'students' taking a test and actually getting a diploma when they graduate. The doctors are some of our younger people who must become familiar with the problems of aging as well as some who are semi-retired. One of our doctor-teachers is 73." It is another beginning.

---

I have a very dear friend who is an inveterate and very typical heavy smoker. It has created a series of problems for her as it does for most smokers, and she suffers from emphysema and all its symptoms, ranging from loss of breath to terrifying coughing fits. And still she smokes, though she has tried to give it up time and time again. Like so many of her friends, I have tried to convince her to do so, sometimes with a smile and at other times in anger. With all her charm, she looks back at me and agrees, and then she says, "If only *my doctor* would scare me and tell me to give it up, I would!"

For my dear old friend, about whom I worry too much, and for all of us in our middle lives, it is time. It is time that we stopped looking to our doctors and time that *we* faced up to the facts of life—and the facts of death. It is time that we stopped idolizing our physicians as deities and dispensers of magic who can cure us with the wave of a prescription pad or scalpel. It is time that we stopped thinking that an unending stream of money can create new technologies that will keep us healthier, if poorer. Whether you like it or not, only *we* can make a dramatic impact in the *maintenance* of our good health. Like it or not! It is about time!

# "Drink Your Milk! It's Good for You!" (Some Thoughts about Nutrition and Exercise)

> *Though I may look old, yet I am strong and lusty...*
> *William Shakespeare:*
> As You Like It

I have a confession to make. I am a supermarket voyeur. Along with you, I push my basket down the endless aisles, awed at the abundance and the variety, seldom able to find a product my first time through. And as I shop I look into the baskets of those who pass, making mental note of the products they buy and what they're planning to have for dinner that evening. Through it all, I generally come to one inflexible conclusion: *I would not want to be invited to most of those homes to dine!*

Frozen TV dinners, packaged puffed, sugar-coated cereals, tissue-textured white bread, frozen lasagna, instant coffee, nondairy chemical creamer, potato chips, corn chips, soda pop, processed meats, ten-pound bags of sugar, plus plenty of animal fat in the form of chopped beef, steak, and bacon. The baskets overflow with colorful boxes, most of them advertised on television and in our consumer magazines. The prices are high, of course, for they include the processing, the advertising campaigns, and chemicals as additives and preservatives.

For a country as rich as ours, as ingeniously inventive when we are forced to be, it is amazing how few people understand that we are essentially a nation of overweight and malnourished individuals, though we consume more food per capita than anyone else in the world. The blame can be apportioned—part of it to ignorance, part to laziness, part to stubbornness, and a great part to a dependence on "experts" who know less about nutrition than we do.

My mother was, perhaps, typical of a generation of immigrants who had struggled very hard and who were determined that their children would never go hungry in a land of plenty. The end result of their hard work, their sacrifice, and their dedication would show up in progeny who were obviously very well fed. I was so skinny as a child that it was painful for me to wear a bathing suit. An early photo, taken at a lakeside resort when I was 13, clearly shows the full number of ribs on a gangling frame, even though the picture has faded after all these years.

For my mother this was a torment, and along with the constant reminders to "Eat!" or "Have a little more," my nemesis was an obese friend named Harold. To coax me onward toward her goals for me, my mother constantly commented, "Look at how nice and healthy Harold looks!" while placing before me custards covered with heavy cream, fat-encrusted steaks and lamb chops, eggs and bacon, chocolate cake, and "rewards" of sugar-coated jelly beans. Of course she meant well and I managed to survive—as we all did—overcooked vegetables with the vitamins drained out along with the water; well-done steak; and a constant diet of cholesterol, saturated fat, and sugar. To top it off, my mother was a terrible cook, and I was one soldier in World War II who did *not* want to come home to "Mom's apple pie"!

Modern technology has taken over where mother left off. We learned to process foods to make it easier to prepare meals for a busy family. Television advertising came along to push the new millenium — instant cereals, enriched foods, chemically preserved, sugar-rich junk food snacks—to make us what Dr. Gay Gaer Luce (*Your Second Life*. Delacorte/Seymour Lawrence, Boston, 1979) calls "the world's proving grounds for cardiac disease," adding that "we are about to become the diabetes capital of the world." For there is evidence that, along with our convenience, we are paying a terrible price. *Our diet may be related to six of the ten leading causes of death in this country.*

This is another area where the media and the corporations of the country well deserve to be on our hit list. The Senate Committee on Nutrition and Human Needs issued a report, signed by Senators George McGovern and Charles Percy, that said in part:

> *Television advertising of edible products, often containing little or no information on nutritional content, shapes early food selection. And most of what is advertised is food with no nutritional value.*

The Ninth International Congress of Nutrition reported in 1972 that "50 percent of the money spent on television food advertising may be negatively related to health . . . items that may be generally characterized as high in fat, cholesterol, sugar, salt, or alcohol."

The medical world is no help to us either. When was the last time your doctor spoke to you about nutrition? When was the last time he or she sat down with you and discussed the alternatives relating to good eating and good health? Probably never, because most doctors know *nothing* about nutrition. It is not taught in the medical colleges because it is basically a preventive science and is not normally directed toward the cure of a particular disease. So when your family physician gives you a loving pat on the shoulder and says, as you leave the office, "I'd like to see you take off five pounds," you have received a full dose of nonadvice because he can't really tell you how to accomplish the feat.

The dieticians and the so-called nutritionists who work in our hospitals are not much better. Have you ever looked carefully at hospital food from the point of view of nourishment? If hospitals were so marvelous in their dietary practices, why would so much sugar-loaded gelatin dessert be served to patients? Dr. Robert Mendelsohn reports on one large Boston hospital that tested surgical patients for protein and calorie malnutrition. Half of them were not getting sufficient amounts of either one "and 25 percent were sufficiently malnourished to lengthen their hospital stay. Other studies have discovered malnutrition in from one-quarter to one-half of the patients in hospitals. *It is a common cause of death among elderly patients.*" (Italics mine.)

Sometimes there is black humor attached to the stories that we read, and we laugh with a little knot in our stomachs at our helplessness and vulnerability. The *Washington Post* sent a reporter to the cafeterias of the government agencies most concerned with health, nutritional protection, and the dissemination of health information: the Food and Drug Administration, the Department of Agriculture, and the Department of Health and Human Services. She found that they specialized in greasy fried meats and potatoes, with little attention paid to fresh fruits, vegetables, and low-calorie foods. They're called "Uncle Sam's fast food emporia."

The Senate Committee reported, "Since the beginning of the century, the composition of the average American diet has changed radically. Complex carbohydrates—fruits, vegetables, and grains—which were the mainstay of the diet now play a minor role. At the same time, fat and sugar consumption have risen to the point where these two dietary elements alone now comprise at least 60 percent of the total caloric intake."

Add to all this the stresses of modern society: the prevalence of smoking and alcohol; the spreading clouds of pollution, even in formerly smog-free cities like Denver and Salt Lake City; the injection of hormones and preservatives, and the ripening of vegetables and fruits by injecting gases, and we begin to see more clearly why all of our nutritional bad habits can have a negative effect on our life expectancy and our resistance to diseases. It becomes even more important to us as we reach middle age. And—rich as our nation is—this is one area where money doesn't seem to save us. In fact, our affluence may be making nutritional matters worse. On a film trip to Vancouver, Canada, this past year, searching for a place to have a quiet dinner with my crew after a hard day's work, we were sent to the "best" restaurant in the city, a place called The Mansion, an elegant and stately house in a quiet section of the city. I scanned the menu for a simple, wholesome selection, something honest, nutritionally acceptable, and unadorned. My search was, of course, in vain. The more expensive the restaurant, the more complex the dishes are likely to be. I found a classic and read it aloud for my companions to hear:

> *Beef, Veal, and Pork topped with Crabmeat . . . Foie Gras*
> *and Artichoke Bottoms, Sauce Bernaise. . .*

My mother would have urged, "Eat, it's good for you. Maybe you'll look like your friend Harold!" But if she were alive today she might very well have laughed with the rest of us. It is never too late to change, and in only the past few years the change has been surprisingly evident almost everywhere we look. Many of us have taken our responsibility to heart and we are finally becoming more aware of what our diets have been doing to our health.

To be sure, it has taken time. The results of drinking hemlock are almost immediate, but the destruction caused by bad diet, smoking, obesity, and lack of exercise may not make itself felt until well into our middle or later years, in the form of chronic disease or premature death. We carry with us a sense of denial—"It can't happen to us"—or we put an inordinate amount of faith in our medical system—"They'll cure us if it does happen." We are a nation that likes a guarantee for everything we buy and do, and there is no guarantee, after all, that a change in health habits will really be good for us. Still, it is amazing to hear that *two-thirds* of the households interviewed in 1979 by the U.S. Department of Agriculture's Economics and Statistics Service reported that they were making dietary changes for reasons of health and proper nutrition! Up to 20 percent had actually reduced their consumption of bacon, sausage, hot dogs, luncheon meats, eggs, beef, and pork, while increasing their intake of poultry, fish, fruits, and vegetables.

This awareness has even extended into the area of insurance. A growing number of companies have begun to offer reduced premiums for their policyholders who do not smoke or drink, who keep their weight down, and who exercise regularly, with an awareness that our bad habits are killing many of us before our time, and are crippling millions of others unnecessarily:

> Obesity is one of the biggest health problems in our society. Dr. Ken Walker was quoted in the *Canadian Medical Association Journal* as saying that the extra pounds equal diabetes and atherosclerosis and, if they were wiped out, "you could fire half the nation's doctors and close half the hospitals."
>
> As little as a 10- to 30-percent weight reduction can lower the blood pressure significantly, the *New England Journal of Medicine* has reported.
>
> Researchers are beginning to discover that lack of correct nutrition may be one of the causes of senility in the aged. And, as we grow older, what we eat may affect our vulnerability to osteoporosis, periodontal disease, anemia, and even starvation.
>
> Coronary disease and strokes can be directly associated with our diets of high fat and high cholesterol as well as the severe effects of smoking, from emphysema to lung cancer, the denials of the cigarette industry notwithstanding.

My father, now 85 years of age, had been smoking since he was 11 years old, sometimes as much as two packs a day. When he reached his 72nd birthday, he gave up his beloved cigarettes, cold turkey, and never once went back to them. The only reason he would give me when I asked him why was, "I just thought I'd feel better." I often think of his answer, and his remarkable willpower after 61 years of inhaling carcinogens, when one of my friends tells me that he or she "would like to quit" but "can't seem to do it."

There is no doubt that we eat too much. As we age, we should be cutting down our intake of food, yet many of us increase the amount we eat. In a number of experiments conducted by the National Institute on Aging, the animals that were given sparse diets lived up to twice as long as those who were on unrestricted feeding. There was a further discovery that curtailing the amount of food also delayed the onset of the chronic diseases associated with old age. I will admit that the experiments took place with species as diverse as chickens and guppies and that the researchers declared that more research was needed, but one conclusion by Dr. Eleanor D. Schlenker brought the subject right back to the area of *our responsibility:* "Many factors determine the health and life span of older people. The individual has little, if any, control of some of these (for example, pollution in the air). But nutrition is one factor which, for most individuals, is subject to a certain amount of choice. Proper nutrition throughout life has been suggested as one of the best means of minimizing degenerative changes as well as increasing life span."

What is proper nutrition? We are just beginning to learn what our grandparents may have instinctively known so many years ago. We are going back to the basics and, as with our physicians, we are beginning to read and to question. I met a neighbor at the little village store just yesterday morning. Eleanor was holding a can at arm's length and reading the label—or, at least, trying to read it without her glasses. I laughed and joined her, for I had also left my glasses back at the house, but since I had longer arms, I could read the information for her. Not too many years ago there was no information on the labels, and, even if there had been, not many of us would have bothered to read the ingredients, the chemical content, or the names of the additives. We might not have been aware of the amount of sugar or salt or noted that "color and freshness are preserved with sodium sulfite and BHA" while the flavor had been enhanced with disodium inosinate and disodium guanylate.

Eleanor also told me of a child she had seen the day before, about seven or eight years old, who had returned a candy bar to the checkout counter because he had read the label and it had "too many strange things in it." A good beginning, indeed, for one so young!

We still can't understand *everything* they tell us and the technical names can be awesome and frightening. But the basic information must be there and, if you are on a restricted diet or you feel as I do that sugar and salt are dangerous to your well-being, at least you have some indication of the amount of the ingredient, though the FDA would like to see the law changed to list the *percentages* used.

Keep in mind, too, that the two most common additives to processed foods—sugar and salt—can also masquerade under other names: *sugar* as corn syrup, dextrose, sucrose, maltose, lactose, fructose, glucose, or invert sugar; *salt* as sodium, sodium chloride, or sodium diacetate.

Naturally the manufacturers will come up with various methods of muddying the waters and the FDA would like to see the law made more precise for such terms as "low cholesterol" or "dietetic." The term "salt-free" may indicate no sodium chloride, but other types of salt may be present.

One of the most misused labeling terms is the word "natural," for it means one thing to some of us and something entirely different to every manufacturer who has discovered that it is the magic word of marketing. It means—to put it bluntly—nothing! Look at the labels on most commercial "natural" products and you will probably see that two of the leading ingredients are "salt" and "sugar." They are, after all, natural, are they not?

For someone such as I, as well as business people all over the country who travel a great deal, another source of nutritional frustration comes in the hotels, motels, and restaurants at which we are obliged to eat. Run by large corporations in many cases, guided by magazines and marketing techniques that emphasize "portion control," specializing in food shipped frozen and microwaved at the last instant, these places offer breakfast, lunch, and dinner that are superb studies in chemistry but are not a balanced diet. (If you want to be thoroughly bored, I have devoted two whole chapters to the subject in a previous book, *Easy Going* [Rodale Press, Emmaus, Pa., 1981].)

I am a latecomer to the world of good nutrition. Though I am no missionary about it, I do believe that these past ten years have seen a tremendous improvement in my health and well-being, and my weight has been easier to keep in check. Thus the food that I encounter on my constant travels can be disappointing, to say the least, as well as a perpetual source of resentment toward the lodging chains and restaurants whose offerings have so lowered the standards of our diets. As a result, I generally take my own picnic meals aboard airplanes, buy fresh fruit and eat it for breakfast in my room, and let the eating establishments know that I am displeased when they serve an array of artificial swill that they would pass off as "gourmet cooking." I am also, occasionally, not pleasant to be with.

We need not perpetuate the same bad habits at home, of course. And more and more magazines—from *Prevention* to *Family Circle*, *Modern Maturity* and *Prime Time*—are publishing articles that can help the consumer find a way through the maze represented by the food industry.

In that sense, the change has been remarkable. With all my complaining, I begin to see a small shaft of light shining through. A pamphlet issued by the U.S. Department of Agriculture in 1972 and revised in 1974 (*Food Guide for Older Folks*) stated that "nutritionists [!] have developed simple food guides to help people make good choices whether they eat at home or eat out." The recipes included frozen dinners, canned and frozen main dishes, processed cheeses, canned corned beef hash, ground meats, dried beef, frankfurters, canned macaroni, bacon, salt pork, beef drippings, and as much as half a teaspoon of salt per recipe!

The pamphlet was eventually withdrawn and a new one was issued just a year or so ago. (*Nutrition and Health*. Superintendent of Documents, U.S. Government Printing Office, Washington, DC 20402.) The change in approach is nothing short of astounding and the new pamphlet lists the seven basic guidelines right on the cover. Gone are the salt pork and the beef drippings. In their place are whole grains, fresh fruits and vegetables—and the avoidance of salt, sugar, cholesterol, and too much alcohol! The seven points contain some very good advice.

# Eat a Variety of Foods

As we get older, we may (and should) cut down on the amount of food we eat. Thus the variety, rather than the amount, of food can give us a well-rounded diet of vitamins, minerals, amino acids (from proteins), essential fatty acids (from vegetable oils), and energy in the form of sufficient calories.

🖉 Fresh fruits and vegetables are an excellent source of vitamins, especially C and A.

🖉 Whole grain products provide B vitamins, iron, and energy, as well as fiber.

🖉 It is no longer believed that "milk is only for babies." Milk and its by-products are excellent sources of high-quality protein, calcium, and vitamins, no matter what our age.

Many of us believe that the biggest waste in the food chain is the rich, fatty meats we love for protein. There are more efficient ways to get whole protein, though I doubt that this advice will ever be listened to in a "steak-crazy" nation. A combination of grains and legumes can make a full protein meal, the equivalent of a large portion of steak, and without the saturated fats. The same protein content can be found in a teaspoon of sunflower seeds!

Be aware of the fact that the processed foods that you buy are changed by the very treatment used in bringing them to your supermarket shelf—generally a diminution in the food value. The RDAs (Recommended Daily Allowances) are also meaningless, for they vary for children, teen-agers and older adults. We are not homogeneous, shot-from-the-same-cannon, like our processed cereals. Some of us have special needs because of illness, the size of our frame, or just plain preference in foods.

# Maintain Ideal Weight

The heavier you are, the greater your chances of developing the chronic disorders that plague our age group. The country is rife with high blood pressure, diabetes, and strokes, much of it the result of excess weight and bad diet. The change that has come about, however, since we were kids is that body weight is no longer based on a rigid height-weight ratio. At last they have taken into consideration the fact that my metabolism may keep me thinner than yours keeps you, and that my frame size and bone structure are different from those of my peers. In fact, some of us can eat large amounts of food and not seem to gain weight, while others merely take a snack once in a while and yet put on too many pounds too quickly.

## Suggested Body Weights

| Height | Men | Women |
|---|---|---|
| (Feet-inches) | (Pounds) | (Pounds) |
| 4'10" | | 92-119 |
| 4'11" | | 94-122 |
| 5'0" | | 96-125 |
| 5'1" | | 99-128 |
| 5'2" | 112-141 | 102-131 |
| 5'3" | 115-144 | 105-134 |
| 5'4" | 118-148 | 108-138 |
| 5'5" | 121-152 | 111-142 |
| 5'6" | 124-156 | 114-146 |
| 5'7" | 128-161 | 118-150 |
| 5'8" | 132-166 | 122-154 |
| 5'9" | 136-170 | 126-158 |
| 5'10" | 140-174 | 130-163 |
| 5'11" | 144-179 | 134-168 |
| 6'0" | 148-184 | 138-173 |
| 6'1" | 152-189 | |
| 6'2" | 156-194 | |
| 6'3" | 160-199 | |
| 6'4" | 164-204 | |

SOURCE: HEW Conference on Obesity.

Don't try to lose weight too rapidly and don't indulge in the crash diets that are the fad these days. Try to lose weight gradually—a pound or two a week. And don't go off too far in the other direction. Severe weight loss can be the cause of everything from hair loss to skin changes, intolerance to colds, constipation, and mental disturbances.

# Avoid Too Much Fat, Saturated Fat, and Cholesterol

Eating foods that contain large amounts of saturated fat and cholesterol tends to elevate the blood cholesterol level in most adults. Though there is still some controversy, evidence seems to point to a high cholesterol level as the prime villain in early heart attack, especially if you suffer from high blood pressure and you smoke.

*▨* Select lean meat, fish, poultry, and dried beans and peas as your sources of protein.

*▨* Moderate your use of eggs and cream, butter, hydrogenated margarines, shortenings, and coconut oil and cut down on your consumption of organ meats such as liver. With regard to coconut oil, you'll notice (if you read the labels) that it is a common ingredient in such items as the nondairy creamers now so prevalent on airplanes and in restaurants. It is loaded with cholesterol!

*▨* Trim the excess fat off meats.

*▨* Broil, roast, bake, or steam rather than fry.

# Eat Foods with Adequate Starch and Fiber

This is an area of much myth, like everything else that seems to affect us as we age. My wife and I were working on a book (*Sheryl and Mel London's Creative Cooking with Grains and Pasta.* Rodale Press, Emmaus, Pa., 1982) that required testing a range of whole grains including oats, barley, rice, amaranth, bulgur, corn, and wheat. It went on for over two years—for breakfast, lunch, dinner, and snacks we had dishes made with grains. The first reaction to all of this from our friends was invariably, "Boy, are you two going to get fat!" We not only did *not* get fat—we felt better and we actually *lost* weight during part of the testing process!

The major sources of energy in our diet are carbohydrates and fats. If, as good nutrition suggests, we lower our intake of fat, then we should increase our caloric intake of carbohydrates. They also help us maintain our weight, since they have about half the calories of fat. However, the *simple* carbohydrates, such as sugar, give us a "quick fix" with calories but provide very little else in the way of nutrition. The *complex* carbohydrates—beans, peas, nuts, fruits, whole grains, and cereals—provide other essential nutrients in addition to the calories. I've read with interest that the sporting world has replaced the familiar pregame or prefight steak with pasta. And so have the long-distance runners.

There is another element that makes the addition of complex carbohydrates important to our nutritional needs. Anthropologists and other scientists have been studying certain African tribes for years, wondering why the incidence of bowel cancer is so low. Their diets are heavy in whole grains, and whole grains add fiber, an element quite low in the average American diet. High fiber content also reduces the symptoms of constipation, diverticulosis, and other modern complaints of "irregularity."

# Avoid Too Much Sugar

I must admit that my diet as a young person, now changed so radically, left me with dreams of jelly beans and Milky Ways. But I paid a price for all the nonstop munching of candies, chocolate, and rich desserts. My teeth have gone through enough reconstructions, excavations, and probing to make them eligible for an archeological foundation grant. The average American consumes about *130 pounds of sugar a year* in coffee, jams, jellies, desserts, soft drinks, cakes, pies, breakfast cereals, catsup, and ice cream, and none of it is nutritionally necessary.

Cutting down for someone like me means an increase in the use of fruits, carrot sticks, nuts, or a piece of whole grain bread as snacks. For anyone in middle age and beyond, the junk foods are better left untouched. I do admit, however, to a little tinge of envy when I see the jar of jelly beans on the desk of an American President.

# Avoid Too Much Sodium

This seems to be the most difficult area in which to abide by the sane rules of nutrition and maintenance of health. We salt our foods almost by rote, both when we cook them and when they reach the table. My wife and I thought that writing a book on grains would necessitate our use of salt, even though we normally do not use it in our house. We felt the same way when we did our book on fish (*The Fish-Lovers' Cookbook.* Rodale Press, Emmaus, Pa., 1980). And both times we were wrong. The clever use of citrus, spices and seasonings, and herbs, and the fact that it is quite possible to learn to enjoy food by tasting its natural flavor, can reduce the amount of salt intake enormously. This morning, for example, just a few moments ago, my wife finished testing her popcorn recipe for the new book. She burst into my office with two large bowls of warm, freshly made popcorn—*without salt*. In my childhood that would have been sacrilege, for anyone in his right mind knew that popped corn must have a large supply of salt. It is just not true—and I suppose that I've come a long way. The snack tasted absolutely superb *au naturel*.

It has been proven time and again that populations with a low sodium intake have less trouble with hypertension and high blood pressure. Japan, for example, uses large amounts of sodium in seasonings such as soy and in pickled condiments and salt-dried fish, and the hypertension rate is astronomical. In America, must of our salt intake is hidden in processed foods—potato chips, pickled products, condiments such as steak sauces, cheese, cured meats, and, yes, commercial popcorn! This is an area where reading the labels can help you determine the salt content and assist you in the reduction of sodium in your diet.

# Take Alcohol in Moderation

The seventh piece of advice given by the USDA and the Department of Health and Human Services is to keep your intake of alcohol moderate if you do drink. Alcoholic beverages are high in calories but very low in nutrition.

Other sources of information are available and an avid reader of any of today's magazines and other literature can quickly become at least a little familiar with the rules of nutrition and good health. They are really quite simple. The National Retired Teachers Association and the American Association of Retired Persons distribute a helpful booklet, *A Guide for Food and Nutrition in Later Years*. It covers supermarket tips, nutrients and their food sources, and special diets, and there is even a small section on how to make eating alone more palatable and enjoyable. (Write: Society for Nutrition Education, 2140 Shattuck Avenue, Suite 1110, Berkeley, CA 94704.)

Dr. Ruth Weg, a physiologist at the Ethel Percy Andrus Gerontology Center, also believes that the patterns of diet and nutrition are more crucial to the well-being of the aging population than they are at any other stage in life and that the ideal or "optimum" diet may be different for us than for younger adults. She has written a book, *Nutrition and the Later Years*, which can be ordered from the Publications Office, Andrus Gerontology Center, USC, University Park, Los Angeles, CA 90007. The price at this writing is $5.50.

Nutrition is still a new and evolving science. Many of the theories are not yet proven and new ones surface every day. It is one reason that the subject of nutrition is so fascinating. The director of the Santa Barbara, California, branch of the American Institute of Family Relations claims that the food we eat is responsible for emotional problems in three out of every four marriages. She reports (in "I'm a Natural," March 1981) that one case is fairly typical. The woman was severely depressed and the man extremely irritable. She advised that the couple stop their consumption of sugar and refined flour and reduce their intake of coffee. "Their relationship turned completely around," she writes. "Her depression lifted. He went from being testy to amiable. They were like honeymooners again."

And don't be surprised, given the new and growing interest in how we eat as well as what we eat, if that old children's nursery rhyme is eventually revised from "Jack Sprat *could* eat no fat. . ." to "Jack Sprat *should* eat no fat. . ." It would be very good advice, indeed!

# The Agony and the Exercise

During the summer months it begins very early in the morning, usually as the sun makes itself felt here on the ocean's edge and my typewriter has yet to compose its first words, a cup of coffee steaming at my elbow. The rhythmic pounding on the boardwalks outside sends a ripple through the beams of the house, sometimes the drumming of two Adidas-clad feet and at other times a couple moving in cadence with their own silent clock. The joggers have begun and they do not stop their exercise no matter how hot it becomes, though the agony is more evident on their faces and in their sweaty bodies as the temperature and the humidity climb.

They are of all ages, shapes, and sizes, men and women and little children being initiated into the cult of masochism. I walk outside and watch with awe the self-flagellation, the punishment, and the misery. But then I do not understand and I suppose I never will. I am not, by nature, a deliberate exerciser and no matter how often the runners explain to me that what I am seeing is actually rapture and ecstasy, the beatitude of exertion, I am among the uninitiated, the unbelievers, the infidels. Suffice it to say that it is exactly one mile from the village store past my house and back again, and so they will be here again tomorrow morning and all through the day.

I have teased and I have been teased through all these years of proclaiming that "exercise is destructive to the muscle tone," for I know that deep, deep down I believe quite the opposite and that, particularly at our age, exercise can do much to preserve our physical fitness and help the body resist disease; delay sluggish circulation; and maintain the strength of our muscles. It is just that I have been lucky and am the end product of a career that has entailed a tremendous amount of physical labor. In short, as Alex Comfort says, "The best exercise is work." And I still do my share of hauling film equipment up mountains at 14,000 feet or a half mile down in a coal mine, constantly pacing while I direct my films, working a 12- to 14-hour day on location, and having a "hyper" personality that does not let fat sit very long on my frame. But I will not, by any stretch of the imagination, punish myself by jogging or playing tennis. There are other alternatives for each of us.

We are, by nature, a sedentary society, unaccustomed to moving very far from our television sets; slaves to the automobile that becomes our seven-league boots to the supermarket, school, our social affairs, and the fast food emporia. There we can sit again and indulge in still more saturated fats and junk-food cholesterol. To top it off, we probably have sat at a desk for 30 years or more.

One day as we hit middle age (whatever that is), we begin to see ourselves with too much bulge in all the wrong places and cellulite overflowing its boundaries, and we decide that it's time to exercise! Violently! Immediately! To make up for all that lost time. Or else we decide that it's not worth the effort and we just let nature take its course. The first choice is dangerous and can bring on cardiac failure. The second choice portends inevitable destruction of the muscle tone and chronic fatigue. As a matter of fact, the National Aeronautics and Space Administration (NASA), in its studies for the space program, found that each three days of total inactivity corresponds to a loss of *one-fifth* of a person's maximum muscle strength!

A group of British doctors voted on the side of *vigorous* exercise when they studied almost 18,000 middle-aged men and found that those who engaged in active and strenuous sports and other fitness exercises had only half the incidence of coronary heart disease as those who did not exercise at all. Those that got heart disease suffered less severe effects and fewer died. In a report in *Lancet*, the British medical journal, they concluded that "vigorous exercise is a natural defense of the body, with a protective effect on the aging heart against ischemia [lack of blood supply] and its consequences."

If we, as middle-aged people, have been exercising strenuously for many years, there is a good chance that we are maintaining our dedication to racquetball or squash, tennis or jogging, or even two rounds of golf each Saturday afternoon. For those of us who have exercised spottily, if at all, there are a number of other ways to keep our bodies fit and limber at 50 or 70 or older.

On my very first trip to Hong Kong back in the early '60s, I looked out of my window one foggy morning and watched in awe as a vast number of people, most of them elderly, moved gracefully through a series of exercises. Each person seemed to move entirely on his own in a rhythmic, predetermined, graceful series of balance shifts, gentle thrusts, and wide arcs. It was my introduction to the remarkable ancient Chinese exercise *t'ai chi ch'uan*. I have watched it many times since then and have photographed it for travel films, and just recently I investigated it still more thoroughly by attending a beginner's class at a local school. It is just one example of what many of us can do to stimulate circulation as we get older, to use grace and balance and rhythm, and to combine an art form with tradition in keeping ourselves more fit and active. There is no need to take up tennis at the age of 50!

The movements of *t'ai chi ch'uan* are simple and elegant and almost create a feeling of ballet in slow motion. *T'ai chi* is often called "swimming in the air." There is no competition, and each participant creates a fluidity based upon his or her own pace. The ages in our class ranged from about 20 up to the early 60s and we wore exactly what we had worn to work that day. No special shoes, no sweat suits, no warm-up, no perspiration, no cool-down, no shower afterward. Best of all, it can be practiced right at home and, as one of the instructors said, "It's such a gentle way to wake the body up, to get all the systems going."

There are many ways to get the system going—and to keep it going at our ages. Dr. Gay Gaer Luce and those in her SAGE (Senior Actualization and Growth Exploration) program in California take a holistic approach to good health as we age. They believe very strongly that physical and emotional health are very much tied together and their program consists of exercises such as *t'ai chi*, yoga, breathing, Sufi dancing, and massage—along with nutrition, chanting, and meditative exercises. It has been so successful that a great many young people have joined what was once a program devoted to the middle-aged and elderly.

In Charleston, West Virginia, there is a remarkable man named Lawrence Frankel, 75 years old, who has designed and developed a physical fitness program that is now being used all over the state in housing complexes, gymnasiums, nursing homes, hospitals, and community centers. It's called Preventicare and it is designed to keep the elderly from "drifting into obsolescence." Mr. Frankel's motto is, "Enforced inactivity in the elderly is death on the installment plan." His students now number more than 3,000, ranging in age from the early 60s to well into the 90s, and though the exercise program is simple— sit-ups, leg lifts, and knee bends—the results have been remarkable and the program is spreading rapidly. Mr. Frankel told an interviewer that nothing makes him more depressed than seeing older people "warehoused" in nursing homes or hospitals, waiting for death in front of the television set!

For some of us exercise can be dancing, programs offered at the local "Y," or just *walking* on our own. At a conference held at the National Institutes of Health in Bethesda, Maryland, in 1977, research participants from the United States, Canada, and Western Europe agreed that walking was the most efficient form of exercise and one that can be safely followed no matter what one's age.

And so I gently withdraw my constant and long-standing maxim that exercise is destructive to the muscle tone. As we enter middle age it is, indeed, more important to us that we stretch more, bend more, and sit less, no matter how we choose to accomplish it.

On this lovely morning, as the sun begins to creep up slowly, I shall take my coffee cup, walk outside my door, and *smile* at the joggers as they gasp their way past my house.

# Part III
# The Changing Face
# of Aging

We are not without our problems, our emotional letdowns, our deep and agonizing questioning of ourselves as we enter into and travel through middle age. My grandmother used to say, "Who ever told you that life would be easy?" And thus my friend Jonathan, just turning 50, is going through the pangs of "Whither go I?" at this time in his life, unable to believe that the years have gone so quickly and that over 100 friends at his birthday party will help remind him that his children are grown and that he has survived quite well through this half century. He will also manage to weather the next decades with ease, once he overcomes the awe that seems to come with the idea of having lived 50 years.

There is no doubt that someone of 20 cannot know what it is like to be 50. I do not say this in a totally negative way, for I am referring as much to the joys of maturity as I am to the problems that are a part of the aging process. Jonathan's reaction is, perhaps, universal in the sense that all of us have felt the onset of middle age as a turning point throughout the generations. Sometimes it strikes as early as the age of 25; for others it comes at 40. Society does little to relieve the shock, as we have seen.

But, in addition to the self-awareness that comes with merely reaching whatever age we consider to be the middle of our lives, there are also the dilemmas that we face merely because we are living in a *particular time*. In that way we are very special, for these are problems that have belonged to no one else. They are very specifically *ours*.

We are the first generations to find ourselves in a world where we are destined to live longer than any who have preceded us. And yet we seem to retire much sooner than our fathers and our grandfathers did. This longer projected period outside the work force brings with it the necessity for more orderly and detailed financial planning, but the ravages of inflation are threatening the secure patterns that we thought we had developed.

To make matters even more threatening, the Social Security system is under attack, though the optimists among us watch it with fingers crossed, knowing that we will somehow survive that problem as we have persisted through so many others in our lives. There may even be cold comfort in the fact that our grandparents, and those who came before them, did not even have a system of retirement benefits, either governmental or private.

But there is one area where this longer expected life span has brought with it a new, serious, and deeply emotional set of complications for those of us in middle age. No other generation has had to face, to the same extent, the realities that have come for so many of us who have elderly parents who are still living.

There are three-generation families and not a few with four generations still alive, sometimes living in the same household. It is not unusual to find a still newer phenomenon—two generations of *retirees* in one family. And thus, just when we feel we have discovered our freedom, the children gone, we hear a cry from another direction. The generation gap reverses and suddenly it is our parents who seem to need help, and they turn inevitably toward us, their middle-aged sons and daughters. In this area *we* are the pioneers, for no one before us has—or could have—written the rulebook by which we can find our way. It is a new responsibility in a life that has held so many changes.

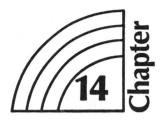

# Well, We Can Always Put Them on the Ice Floes

> *Cast me not off in time of old age; Forsake me not when my strength faileth.*
>
> Psalms 71:9

The books and the advice came too late to be of any help to us. We were in the beginnings of an awareness of the problem and an occasional newspaper article told us that we were not alone. Even now, so many years later, I am not quite certain how we might have approached things differently. I have learned, however, that my solution to the situation was quite wrong; that my wife, Sheryl, in her stubbornness, was far ahead of her time.

Only this past year, almost ten years after the problem had surfaced and five years after my mother-in-law, Kitty, had died, I watched Dr. Stephen Z. Cohen, author of *The Other Generation Gap* (Paperback. Warner Books, New York, 1978), on the tape of a television program and I nodded in mute agreement as he told the interviewer:

> *People have always had parents who have grown old and have needed assistance, but what's special in our country*

133

*today is that so many more people are living to an advanced old age. We now have approximately 23 million people in the country who are over age 65, and the prospect is that many more will achieve 70, 80, 90 years of age. Living that long poses many problems for the older person and for the children. There's the prospect of living with a variety of chronic illnesses and that means that people are going to turn to their children most frequently. Unfortunately, there has been very little discussion of these problems in the country.*

Kitty's slow and agonizing decline took place over a period of five years, beginning when she was 80. For the first three of those years the chronic diseases seemed to vie with one another to make themselves known. Added to the rapidly diminishing eyesight caused by glaucoma, the symptoms of Alzheimer's disease (senility) had begun to make themselves felt, from being unable to choose her own clothing—wearing a sweater as a hat—to the mismatched pieces of silverware placed on the table before her dinner—two knives on one side of the plate, a fork, a knife, and a tablespoon on the other. Her conversations were vivid remembrances of minute details that occurred in 1934, but she could barely recall what she had had for lunch two hours before. That most remarkable computer, the brain, had begun to accept nothing new while continuing to function exquisitely in the past.

To this day I am not quite certain that the symptoms of senility, and of the Parkinson's disease that later struck her, were not the result of the side effects of Thorazine and the other drugs that had been prescribed for her. Whatever the cause, the symptoms were there and the degeneration continued. The generations were reversing, and on that tape so many years later, Dr. Cohen described it all quite accurately:

*There is an expectation, a long-standing tradition in our culture, that somehow we are required to take care of elderly parents. It dates back to the commandment, "Honor thy father and thy mother." Yet, for many people, the fulfillment of that prescription is very difficult. And, for many middle-aged people, the caring for an older person over a long period of time poses terrible problems. For some, the relationship that existed over a period of time becomes strained and painful for both parties.*

Dr. Cohen might well have added, "and painful or destructive to the marriages of the middle-aged children." There are new decisions to be made, the normal expectancy that it might all disappear in time, knowing full well that it will not. There are the differences of opinion, the guilts and the anxieties of commitment, the pressures, and the anticipations of the months, the years to come.

Kitty was of her generation, just as we are of ours and our children reflect the particular virtues and imperfections of theirs. Outwardly frail, with a cameolike beauty that remained with her until the day she died, her luminescence gave a sense of delicacy and helplessness that covered a great reservoir of strength and determination. Her credo, as expressed to us when we were first married and we told her that we had decided not to have children, was, "Who will take care of you when you're old?"

By the end of the third year, when she was 82, the occasional observation of Kitty's daily life, the telephone calls several times a day to see that she did not turn on the gas stove and leave it unattended, had become a constant routine of supervision. She still lived in her apartment only a block away, but now the trips that Sheryl made became more frequent, the daily exercise walks to the park more frustrating and time-consuming. The diseases continued their inexorable march and the drug therapy added to the toll, making Kitty still more dependent, still more disoriented, and more in need of constant attention.

To make matters still worse, Sheryl's older sister, now in Florida and retired, was unable to share the burden. She had contracted cancer and was to undergo a mastectomy. The responsibility fell with all its weight on one person, Sheryl. Since that time, I have learned that this is quite common. One child bears the cross and it is most often a daughter.

After that third year my reaction was a simple, American, knee-jerk response—possibly the answer that many readers will have thought of as this chapter unfolds. It is the first, the almost immediate, answer in our country to the problems of aging and chronic disease: "Put her in a nursing home!"

Sheryl adamantly refused. "I wouldn't put my dog in a kennel," she retorted. "I certainly am not going to put my mother in a nursing home." There had to be a way, she firmly maintained, to handle the problem without taking Kitty from familiar surroundings and isolating her; to let her retain her dignity, and to give her the kind of care and consideration that is so sorely lacking in America's geriatric wards.

I had worked in nursing homes and in the chronic disease wards as a filmmaker and I had seen the emotionless, empty, deadly stares of the patients who sat interminably doing nothing. I had seen the half-hearted attempts at "arts and crafts" and the shocking conditions that exist even in the best of the homes. I had come back from film trips emotionally exhausted and unable to get the images from my mind, all of them as indelibly implanted as they had been on the film we'd shot. And yet, when faced with the rapid deterioration, the physical and mental retrogression, of my own mother-in-law, I immediately thought of quarantine, the surgical removal of the patient from active society.

It was a time when black humor became rampant as the difficulties mounted. I recalled the wonderful book about Eskimos that I read when I was still a teen-ager. The elders of the community, no longer able to function in an environment that was now hostile and threatening, no longer able to chew and soften walrus hides with teeth that were worn to the gums, were put on the ice floes to drift outward into the Arctic Sea, their fate accepted by them and by the younger members of the community, who would one day also ride the ice floes to their destiny. I remember, too, reading of the anxious daughter of one of the elders who shouted to her father, "Jump into the water, father, and put your head under. It will be easier that way!"

Over the next two years, Kitty's condition deteriorated even more rapidly, and I learned much about caring and responsibility and devotion as I watched Sheryl handle it. The resolve that the mother had shown so often in her lifetime was obviously passed on to her younger daughter through the family genes, for Sheryl was quite determined to see it through and to find help somehow. It was not, by any means, easy. The drug intake and the rapid physical deterioration continued, finally making Kitty bedridden and incontinent. She was blind. She took very little food. The mother had become a child, helpless and swathed in diapers, yet her daughter did not yield even an inch.

She actually found help. She determinedly pursued her original intent that her mother would not be left to die in a strange and foreign place. She probed the community social services, explored by telephone bureaucratic mazes of nonanswers, noninformation, misinformation, and double talk. Some of her most important leads came from a remarkable ophthalmologist, Dr. Ralph Salatino, whom we still see and revere today as doctor and friend. He suggested organizations that were specifically designed to help the legally blind. From them, other bits of information surfaced. Sheryl discovered that there *are* people and organizations that not only listen, but can move mountains if they choose. There are an increasing number of community resources that can and do assist middle-aged children in caring for their older parents.

Since Kitty was legally blind, she was entitled to additional money with which to live. There were medical and social programs that would help in the purchase of the horribly expensive drugs, the food supplements, and even the medical paraphernalia that began to fill her room. The costs of all this care are no small matter if the children are forced to pay for the help. With today's medical costs soaring, any family might be financially destitute within months. It is a consideration and a very critical one. Were it not for the programs that Sheryl uncovered, we would have been economically devastated, stripped of our savings. I have nightmares when I think of an administration in Washington that speaks of cutting just these programs, unable to understand that they may well represent salvation for the middle class as well as the poor of our country.

The final and most critical help came from the homemaker program of our city. It provided a remarkable woman named Ivy Thomas, who cared for her bedridden patient for over a year, and she was with her until the moment she died at 4 o'clock on a fall afternoon.

It is five years since that terrible time, and Sheryl has not changed her mind. She would do it again. *My* solution would not have worked, for this way Sheryl is at peace with herself, without guilt, knowing that she did the best she possibly could. The situation, of course, was an extreme one, and I recount it here as only one example of what can happen as our parents age. Luckily it is not the typical case, but it made me search deeply for the reasons behind my reactions.

Like many of my middle-aged peers, I am the victim of still another set of myths about the aged, another series of social lies that distort our thinking when the problems of elderly parents become a personal burden of conscience. It is no small comfort to me to learn that I am not alone, that 75 percent of all nursing students polled in a recent study thought that almost all people over 65 were residing in nursing homes! When young psychologists were asked about it, 35 percent thought exactly the same thing. In fact, the actual statistic is astoundingly low—only *4 to 5 percent* of the elderly are institutionalized! Even then it is usually a last resort—these are older people without families, immigrants who came to this country alone and who never married, widows and widowers without other means of family support.

In spite of what we think, it turns out that our middle-aged brothers and sisters do *not* heartlessly dump their parents, abandoning them to an impersonal end. In fact, almost *80 percent* of the people over 65 in our country are living with someone else, not necessarily their children, and usually right in the communities in which they have *always* lived! And the people who do retire to age-segregated communities, such as Leisure World, do so voluntarily. Older Americans are not so likely to live with their children or to receive financial help from them as they once were. Even here the world of aging is undergoing tremendous changes.

In a report published by the Department of Health and Human Services, Prof. Alvin Schorr of Case Western Reserve University concluded that only one-sixth of elderly parents live with their children, compared with one-third in 1952. In addition, 5 to 10 percent received financial assistance from their children in 1961, while *only 2 to 3 percent* do so now. There have been studies, in fact, that show that more cash assistance flows *downward* from older parents to their middle-aged children and grandchildren than in the opposite direction!

Still, there is no doubt that this new resettling of the generations is creating problems. As Dr. Cohen says, "Where the relationships have been close and the children and parents have been together for a long time, those children respond naturally to the needs of the parents. But where there has been a considerable amount of emotional distance or where the children live a thousand miles away, this is a major problem."

The demands of the aging parent may be minimal—merely a request that we be more available or supportive—or they may be as extreme as Kitty's and the tyranny of helplessness. But it is all so unexpected and it is not easy, certainly. There is guilt on both sides of the generation gap. And there is no small amount of anger and resentment on the part of the children, who thought they could finally see the light in their own careers, their own dreams of relaxation and recreation, only to find themselves confronted by the new demands of their parents.

Except for the small percentage of very real physical or chronic problems, it is possible that, in many instances and within the normal cycle of the aging process, *it is we, the children, who help create the situation in which the parents become dependent upon us.*

The physical changes of aging are almost predictable. There are changes in hearing—it took my father almost ten years to admit that a hearing aid might help. Our eyesight certainly does not improve with age—how many of us will read this book while wearing glasses? There is a slowing down of many life processes as we age—we don't move quite so quickly, we breathe more rapidly with physical exertion, we become more deliberate in our movements. The children watch anxiously and are all too ready to rush in, to intervene.

The slight case of forgetfulness, passed over when it occurs in youngsters, becomes cause for worry about creeping senility in our parents. We are so quick to use the word. I do it myself. Senility. More accurately, senile dementia, or Alzheimer's disease, named for the doctor who isolated it. It is part of another damaging myth that creates unnecessary anxiety and anguish. "I believe more people fear senility, fear growing old and losing their minds and being put away than fear cancer," said Dr. Robert Butler, director of the National Institute on Aging. It is just this fear that creates our own foreboding as we see our aging parents become more forgetful, and we too rapidly step in to "help." Likewise, our doctors are too quick to diagnose a condition that might well be caused by a vast array of other factors.

Only a minority of the very old show signs of forgetfulness and confusion, often the harmless and normal effects of the body slowing down. For others, it can be caused by the stress of retirement; loss of income; bereavement; depression; diseases of the heart, thyroid, or lungs; liver infections; nutritional deficiency; or the cocktail mix of drugs given too freely to control the aging mind.

Even discounting illness and imagined disorders, we are too quick to interfere with the agenda and the independence of our parents' lives, just as our children try to do with us. Think of our response when one of our parents, perhaps widowed for ten or more years, decides to remarry at the age of 75 or 80! A thousand reactions and emotional depths are suddenly thrust upon us, the middle-aged children. I have observed resentment and jealousy, feelings of loss, anger at financial arrangements, and discomfort at the reemergence of romantic and sexual activity. I have even heard this phenomenon described by one woman as a "traumatic nightmare!"

Yet it is just this kind of *independence* that the aging parent so desperately needs. It is the continued functioning of parents on their own that helps maintain their strengths and their abilities, making them less dependent upon their children. "Most people can be helped with occasional intervention in their lives," Dr. Cohen says. "Gerontologists are coming to see that the independence of the parent, the continued functioning as much as possible on his or her own, is far better than putting them in a nursing home or moving them into the children's home. With occasional help, they may be able to continue functioning independently for a longer period of time."

Most of our parents need only occasional help. And, if there is no single solution for every family problem, there *is* one universal word to keep in mind—*independence*. We are, the author included, too quick to want to infantilize our parents the moment they show signs of aging or of needing a small amount of help in keeping their self-sufficiency and their dignity. At the same time that *we* resent being judged by our chronological ages, we begin to do the very same thing to them, knowing full well that there are people in their 80s and even their 90s who are active and mentally alert: who remain in the community as participating citizens until their deaths.

For those of our parents who begin to fail physically, the help needed is frequently minimal. It is a good idea to step back and analyze what can be done before rushing in and making a decision that requires that they move in with us or that we isolate them in a nursing facility. There are aging men and women who need only an occasional bit of help from a friend, a neighbor, or from us, and with that help can remain active right where they live. Being in touch with life is a more effective solution than the isolation we sometimes decree for them. It is interesting to note that more than 5 million people over the age of 65—over 20 percent of that segment of the population—have no children, and yet most of that group are *not* institutionalized.

In spite of my fears about administrations in Washington that seem never to be aware of the problems of the middle class, I observe with interest that there are some enlightened legislators who are beginning to notice that even a minimal amount of care in the homes of the elderly, rather than complete care in institutions, might well stop the enormous escalation of health care costs. I also note that eight bipartisan senators did not forget the human elements in a new piece of legislation designed primarily to stem the hemorrhage of money that accompanies our medical costs.

Senator Bill Bradley commented, "Individuals placed in institutions suffer a variety of costs. They are uprooted from their homes; they are severed from normal contact with their family, friends, and community. They experience a serious loss of personal dignity and independence." The statistics vary. The Senate has found that between 10 and 20 percent of the 1.5 million Americans in nursing homes could live in their own homes if they had adequate help. The Gray Panthers consider the entire situation a scandal and claim that *40 percent* of the people in nursing facilities are capable of being on their own, given some help from the community.

If your family situation is one in which your parents are still living but the need for help seems to be growing, it might be wise to investigate the assistance available right in your community before making any drastic decisions or feeling that the world is coming to an end. Having gone through much of it myself, I know the feelings of panic mixed with unease as one turns toward a vast maze of hoped-for solutions. It is quite possible that your parents will never have to live in your home. It is more than probable that you will never have to make the decision even to look at a nursing facility.

A good place to begin is with Dr. Cohen's excellent book, *The Other Generation Gap.* I wish it had been written before the years of our own family hardships. I like it best because Dr. Cohen believes that a great part of the solution is in *understanding* the process of aging, as well as assessing our own emotional reactions to the new family problems of our generation. Most important of all, Dr. Cohen believes that there is much that we can do to prolong the independence of our parents, utilizing both our own efforts and the help given by community organizations such as Meals-on-Wheels and the visiting nurse service.

Beginning about 1975, many other books have been written on the very same subject, and from each of them there is something to be learned before you begin the long process of discussion with your family, the endless telephone calls, and the probing that will eventually help you to find your own solutions.

*When Your Parents Grow Old,* by Jane Otten and Florence D. Shelley (Funk & Wagnalls, New York, 1976), is valuable as a basic resource book. In the beginning realization that a severe parental problem is arising, we all need some new ideas. The names of organizations blur into a meaningless alphabet, and what holds for one state or community may not be available in another. This book contains an appendix on "Where to Write," including Federal Government Programs, Consumer Information, Crime Prevention, Health, Housing (both city and rural), Legal and Financial Management, Nursing Home Information, and Volunteer Programs. A second appendix lists organizations to which you might turn for information and help, including National Organizations for Older People, National Health Organizations, Home Care, and Government Agencies on Aging for each state in the country.

*You and Your Aging Parent,* by Barbara Silverstone and Helen Kandel Hyman (Pantheon Books, New York, 1976) covers much the same psychological and emotional ground as the others, including guilt, disruption, and facing up to the reality of the situation. It explores what the authors call "the endless possibilities" that are available to those aged 65 and over. For our parents, as well as for us, they point out that by knowing the alternatives, there may be less reason to dread these years. One appendix lists the state offices on aging plus informational and referral services across the country. A second section gives addresses under Homemaker-Home Health Aid Services, Family Service Agencies in the United States and Canada, Volunteer Service Organizations, and Opportunities for Paid Employment.

If your parents have begun to develop the chronic diseases that often accompany the aging process, a book by Lawrence Galton (*Don't Give Up on an Aging Parent*. Crown, New York, 1975) may give you a better understanding of just what medical science has learned about everything from arthritis to memory loss. Galton calls them the "so-called illnesses of the aged" and is a great believer (along with the author) that doctors practice what he calls "condescension medicine"— what can you expect when the patient is getting older?

In my research I discovered one more book that may well give you some ideas on where to turn for advice. *Handbook of Human Services for Older Persons* by Monica Bychowski Holmes and Douglas Holmes (Human Sciences Press, New York, 1979) provides an overview of information and referral services; multipurpose senior centers; homemaker and home health agencies; legal, residential repair, employment, and day care services; and nursing home advocacy. It is more technical than the others and each chapter has been written by a different author involved with social welfare and community work, but it is listed here as still another resource that may be of help to you.

In addition, today's magazines and even the television documentary programs have begun to concern themselves with the problems of middle-aged children with elderly parents. My files are crowded with new ideas, new approaches, new thinking—all designed to keep the elderly independent and active instead of incarcerated in institutions.

The Gray Panthers have encouraged and pioneered intergenerational living, where young and old share living quarters. As a matter of fact, Maggie Kuhn shares just such a house in Philadelphia with younger people, most of them about the age of 30. The occupants learn from one another and give mutual help in a group setting. The idea is spreading.

In California a small organization called Housing Alternatives for Seniors provides a "matchmaking" service for people like our parents who should no longer live alone, or who don't want to live by themselves after widowhood. Actually the founders prefer to call it a service that finds "roommates," compatible partners for strong, elderly people who want companionship and who want to retain their independent life style.

There are programs across the country that have been designed especially for people like us. For example, support groups have been formed in almost every state to help us distinguish between the actuality of Alzheimer's disease and the myths about senile dementia. There are programs at the Andrus Gerontology Center in California, at Duke University, in Seattle, in Denver, and in New York. The most important contribution, I think, is that the organization (called Alzheimer's Disease and Related Disorders Association) deals with the actual *disease* rather than the folklore that has made us think of it as a natural consequence of aging. There are 25 chapters around the country and you can write for information to ADRDA at 292 Madison Avenue, New York, NY 10017. Enclose a legal-sized, stamped, self-addressed envelope.

In a recent issue of the magazine *Prime Time,* I read of still another organization that was formed to provide psychological support to middle-aged children with aging parents. It's called Children with Aging Parents (CAPS) and it was started in Los Angeles by the National Council of Jewish Women. It is but one of a growing number of self-help groups and its founders noted that usually our first response to any sign of aging in our parents is to assume they are on the road to inevitable disintegration. "The result," they say, "is that children begin to infantilize their parents. 'Dad, you can't drive the car anymore.' 'Mom, you can't cook in the kitchen because you forgot to turn off the stove once.' Although often done out of the best of motives, the effects are still pernicious." They believe, as I do, that though the parents may be losing some physical abilities, it doesn't make them totally disabled or incompetent.

There are programs designed to help the children of parents who have had to move in with them by giving them a day off or a weekend away from the emotional and physical burdens. Programs that provide transportation for the elderly to the clinic or the doctor. Programs for mutual support. Programs for recreational activities. A national program administered by ACTION provides about 700 local offices throughout the country with about 275,000 volunteers who serve in community agencies and organizations. It's called RSVP, Retired Senior Volunteer Program, and it has a dual purpose: it helps to enrich the lives of older people by giving them the satisfaction of helping others and it also helps local agencies to meet the needs of their communities.

There are more, so many more, which can and do help. I found a fascinating program in New York, run by the Community Service Society and called the Natural Supports Program, which is designed to help families and individuals who are caring for an older person. In addition to providing a necessary forum where moral support and information can be exchanged, it offers the friends and relatives of the aging up-to-date information about agencies and the benefits to which our parents may be legally entitled. It is a growing supplement to, rather than a substitute for, our responsibilities in a burgeoning awareness of a problem which will continue to increase in the coming years.

I suppose I might say, "I wish I had known." But that would be 20-20 hindsight. This morning, at a hurried breakfast with Sheryl, anxious to get back to tell as much as I could in this space that is, unfortunately, limited, I spoke of the research I had done, the people to whom I had spoken, the feeling that there was, indeed, help available to my brothers and sisters. And she asked, "If you had known all this ten years ago, would you still have insisted upon the solution of a nursing home?"

I might easily have answered, "No, of course not." But I must honestly say that I do not know. Though I *think* that I am now enlightened, it is difficult for me to go back to those days of depression and anguish and the tensions in our marriage created by a degenerating, incontinent patient, even though my wife was the one who bore the responsibilities. Most of the people I have known who finally decided to place their parents in a nursing facility have lived for the rest of their lives with guilt and a feeling of having let their parents down when they needed them most. Possibly that would have been my emotional heritage too. I cannot answer it now.

My wife lives with the feeling that she did what she could and her conscience is clear. I cannot, in addition, advise anyone to make the decision for or against a nursing home. So much is at stake and there are so many mitigating circumstances—financial, social, geographic, physical, and varying degrees of family closeness. I, who would have made just such a decision some years back, would not dare pontificate or proselytize at this point in my life.

There is much information now available if you and your family should decide on a nursing home as a last resort. In Dr. Cohen's book, a useful pamphlet issued by the National Retired Teachers Association, a comprehensive Citizens Action Guide published by the Gray Panthers, and numerous other publications, much has been written about evaluating and selecting a nursing home. And all the publications carry negative warnings and stories of isolation and loneliness.

The problem is not, by any means, a hopeless one. We tend to forget that so very many of our parents are still quite active in their 70s and 80s and beyond. I see them all in my own little community. The neighbor's 80-year-old grandfather, just out of the hospital after a gall bladder operation and on his bicycle the very next day! The 70-year-old parachute jumper. The surf fishermen who stand beside me in the ocean in the autumn, some of them in their mid-80s, all of them out-fishing me, a mere stripling of a lad. As we resent being made "old" before our time, so do they. And as the physical strengths begin to disappear gradually, our support is so very much needed *before* we scream "senility" and "put them in a nursing home!" I speak as much to myself as I do to you. I have not proven, after all, to be a paragon of clearheadedness and logic.

Summing up is difficult, to say the least, because each family's personality, each situation, is so different from mine or those of my (or your) friends and neighbors. The Colonial Penn Group asked Dr. Cohen to condense his thinking and his advice. In a booklet called *Bridging the Other Generation Gap* (available free from Colonial Penn Group, Inc., 5 Penn Center Plaza, Philadelphia, PA 19181), he concludes with some points to remember and I reprint them here with permission:

## If You Are an Older Parent:

🌈 Remain as independent as you can.
🌈 Keep active and involved with others. Remember, use it or lose it.
🌈 Your children are adults—don't try to take over their lives.
🌈 Worrying brings you little—talk over your concerns with your children or a close friend.
🌈 Your children are not the only ones able to help you manage.
🌈 Getting help from a social worker or counselor is a sign of strength, not weakness.

## If You Are a Middle-Aged Child:

🌈 Encourage your parents to remain as independent as possible.
🌈 "Doing for" your parents can make them dependent—help them to do for themselves.

⬡ Your parents are adults—don't expect to change them to suit you.

⬡ More open discussion of problems with your parents can usually relieve the tension that comes from not knowing what the trouble is.

⬡ Other relatives and friends may be more than pleased to help out with your parent.

⬡ More and more professionals are available to help you and your parents. Use them.

There is another thing to keep in mind, if you will. The "view from there" may be quite different from the "view from here." What is it like for *our parents* to look back at us from their point of view? What is their reaction if we rush in too quickly to help when no help is asked for or, on the other hand, when we are not there quickly enough when they feel they need us? Their answers can sometimes surprise us, even make us laugh if we listen. In an ad for the Colonial Penn Group there appeared part of a letter from a California woman who might well have answered for many of our parents. "The real shocker in aging," she wrote, "is seeing one's darling babies tottering around as white-thatched old codgers. I'm 88 and I feel exactly the same as I felt at 18. *It's my darned children that depress me!*"

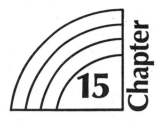

# "Help! I'm a Prisoner in Paradise!"

> *Two weeks is about the ideal length of time to retire.*
>
> *Dr. Alex Comfort*

$M$y father had worked since he was 11 years old—and for 72 years more he knew nothing *but* hard work. As a young man of 17, part of an immigrant family living on New York's Lower East Side, he supported his mother, stepfather, and their assorted progeny by becoming a professional boxer at $5 a fight ($15 for the main event). He slept on three wooden kitchen chairs pulled together for the night on the fifth floor of a walk-up tenement on Rivington Street.

It was expected; a natural period in the process of growing up and he never spoke of it in later years. In fact, I only knew of his early career when I happened to read a sports column written by Jimmy Cannon, in which he longed for the early days of the superb clubhouse fighters. There, among the list of names, was that of my father. He had been known as "Kid" London!

Through seven decades he knew very little but his work and the support of a family. During the Depression, I remember that we saw 147 little of him as he struggled with a tiny garment manufacturing business for 18 to 20 hours a day, still managing to send us to the mountains during the summer to get us away from the city heat, while he stayed behind to keep the struggling business afloat.

Even when the economic situation eased somewhat, and he was a respected and well-paid production manager in the garment trade, he knew very little but work. For a while he owned a dude ranch and, when he went there on weekends, he rode and played as hard as he had worked during the week. At the age of 75 he was still entering 4-H club horseback-riding contests, while complaining of the indignity of having to be helped into the saddle!

Two years ago, when he was 83, he finally retired, forced to slow down by the natural onset of physical aging. It must have been a terribly difficult, though necessary, decision. He had remained fairly active almost until the time he decided to retire. He had walked the 20 blocks to work, had communed with the retired executives, the hangers-on, and the drifters who sat in Washington Square Park, had frequented the restaurants that dot the city, and then suddenly decided that the cold weather, the gradual loss of hearing, and the muscles that no longer obeyed as quickly as they once did had forced him to make the ultimate decision. He and my stepmother moved down where the palm trees wave in a tropical sun, where oranges and avocadoes, mangoes and lemons are outside the door for the picking, and where the seductive blue water of the swimming pool flickers just a few steps from the living room door.

It is an understatement to say that my father is miserable. The air in Florida is often dripping with humidity; the house they purchased, with the fruit trees outside, is isolated, and neither of them drives. The swimming pool is covered with falling leaves and is constantly in need of care. And the man who worked only at work all his life has no other real interests. The motor is idling. But his sense of humor and his quick mind are still with him and, when I telephone to ask how he is, I hear a plaintive wail come back over the long-distance lines, *"Help! I'm a prisoner in Paradise!"*

*I* will never retire. But that's what my father said. I will *never* retire. But I am seduced by the word as my father was seduced by the tropical marsh that passes for his retirement cloister. I will never *retire*. The radio plays the commercial for a large brokerage concern; "Thank you, Paine Webber, I've never been thrifty. Thank you, Paine Webber, I'm retired at 50." I mutter, "poor guy," and go back to my writing.

The newspaper communicates its own urging and promises to me in a full-page ad for a retirement village that says, "Leisure Knoll is us." And it goes on to urge: "Maybe it's you, too. It makes you glad you're 55." Well, it isn't *me*. And maybe it's not even *you*. But, as we move into our middle years, the word "retire" suddenly seems to spring to life and to be forced upon us by the media, by our corporations, and even by our own thoughts. Retire! The Golden Years. The Leisure Years. Sitting back on our asses and reaping all the rewards to which we are entitled. Isolated in age-segregated societies "with dawn-to-dusk roving patrols that assure our peace of mind," making certain that nothing gets in, or possibly that we don't get out. That is my own hostile view.

But there is another side. There are people who actually want to retire, and a large proportion are choosing ages as early as 50 or 55. For some it is a normal, looked-for, expected event, and surveys have shown that up to 70 percent are perfectly content with their retirement lives *if proper planning takes place* in the preretirement years! It is time to look hard at just what the word really means to each of us. My damnation may well be your salvation, while your dream may well be my nightmare.

We can all give silent thanks to Chancellor Otto von Bismarck of Germany for pulling the magic figure of 65 out of his pointed steel helmet back in 1881. In those days very few people lived past the age of 65, so it stood to reason that Bismarck—no fool he—would choose that age at which to reward his workers with the world's first social security program. After all, if just a few Germans lived past that age, the treasury wouldn't have to deliver too many marks to the pensioners. It was as good a number as any, and it has stayed with Western society ever since, eventually being adopted by our legislators back in the '30s when our own Social Security system was being developed.

But, along with an enlightened social program (now under attack from so many legislative directions), there came a societal expectation of planned obsolescence, very much as with electric appliances. Ready or not, we are expected to retire. It is taken for granted that we are suddenly unable to assume the same responsibilities, function as efficiently in our workplace or within the family unit, or keep our places in the "real" world of active, vital human beings as we did for so many years. Even the synonyms for this vaunted, supposedly idyllic "afterlife" give lie to the broken promises of society. My favorite desk book, *The Synonym Finder* (J. I. Rodale. Rodale Press, Emmaus, Pa., 1979) is a treasure trove of depressing words to describe the state of retirement:

"withdrawal, removal, retreat, departure, shelved, rejected, castaway, discarded." Then my eye is drawn to the words used for machinery: "throw out, scrap, junk, abandon use of, withdraw from service, disuse"!

Maggie Kuhn puts it well, as always. "We've been brain-damaged by a society that believes old age is a disease. When we turn 65, we're trashed. . . . When I travel to my home from the airport in Philadelphia, I pass a junkyard where old cars are left to rust on a heap and then they're finally smashed by a society that wants everything shiny and new. America does the same thing to people."

For centuries American corporations have been handmaidens of the idea of forced retirement, holding out the inviting picture of a life of leisure amidst sun-drenched horizons—demanding in return, for 30 years or more, the corporate attributes of conformity, productivity, performance (known as the bottom line), and subordination of personal life to the corporation's needs. In spite of the fact that older workers have consistently been found to be among the most productive, the most talented, reliable, and adaptable, not to mention among the most loyal, millions of us have been forced into another type of unemployment, this one dictated by the calendar. For, make no mistake about it, as Alex Comfort so rightly declares, retirement is nothing more than unemployment and those of us who are unprepared for it will suffer the consequences just as surely as do minority teen-agers who *want* to work but who find all doors closed to them.

Of course, I have seen situations in which I would be most anxious to retire, had I been unfortunate enough to be working for 30 years in the impossible conditions of some of America's factories. The aluminum and steel industries boast assembly lines where the heat rises to over 150°F and the outside temperature of a summer day in Chicago seems cool at 95! Workers change shifts at the machines every 20 minutes and, in one aluminum plant where they recycle scrap, the lens cap on our camera melted as we were photographing the molten metal being poured into ingots!

The closed, noisy, dust-ridden cotton mills of the South, the dangerous working conditions of so many assembly lines, the lethal dangers of the chemical and asbestos industries would make me *run* toward retirement to escape from a world that paid me well but that made me hate my job. Any alternative would be better than the job situations I've described, even sitting in front of a television set, beer in hand, letting my mind and my body slowly distintegrate.

For the rest of us, possibly for relatively few, the notion of leisure holds little meaning, especially if it is translated into doing nothing. There are millions of us who do not want to retire, either forcibly or voluntarily. There are many of us who will retire only to begin new careers, and I have devoted an entire chapter to this phenomenon. In the Harris study on aging it was found that the notion of leisure actually has less relevance among older people than it does among the young in our country; that retirement has more appeal for the young than for the middle-aged and the old! It is no surprise to find out that most of us *want* to remain active, in spite of the societal myth that retirement means almost total withdrawal from life.

Thus, in a time when one trend seems to indicate that more and more of us are deciding on early retirement, an opposite trend is taking us toward even later retirement than before, and both options exist side by side even though they seem to conflict philosophically.

In the first place, some of us who had planned to retire at an early age have found that the increased rate of inflation will not allow us the choice. Most corporate pension plans have just not kept pace with the cost of living, though Social Security and the governmental pension plans have built-in escalators based upon the inflation rate. But even some of us who feel that the nest egg is sufficient to allow us to stop working or to change direction are very much aware of the hazards inherent in the soaring costs of medical and hospital care; the future threatens to make these costs an impossible financial burden for those of us who live on a fixed income. It is even affecting the thinking of the younger generations, and there is a projection that many of the workers in the 35-to-40 age group today may have to think of retirement no earlier than age 70 or 75 if they hope to live comfortably!

But this trend toward later retirement also has its positive side, and I return to those of us who do not want to become inactive. On January 1, 1979, the new age-discrimination law went into effect; it dictates that a worker cannot be retired forcibly until the age of 70, rather than 65 as before.

At the same time America's companies are slowly finding that older workers are a great, untapped repository of know-how and experience. Our health is much better than it has ever been and we actually have better attendance and work records than our younger counterparts. But still another factor has made the companies more aware of just how valuable we are and has made them more receptive to delaying the retirement of older workers. The declining birth rate has made fewer and fewer younger workers available and ready to move up to positions in supervision and management. The corporate world is, first of all, a pragmatic one and, however youth-oriented it is, empty places on the corporate ladder mean less productivity. So we are slowly being discovered. But, given the chance, our companies run true to form. When I look at the history of age-discrimination, I cast a wary eye again at a government that wants to reduce its surveillance of age and sex bias in industry. The record has not been a good one overall.

Standard Oil of California, for example, decided to reduce its work force and it laid off 160 employees, all selected on the basis of age. In a suit in a federal court the company was forced to rehire 120 workers and pay almost $2 million in back pay, with reinstatement in the pension and stock-purchase plans as well as insurance coverage. Without federal law there would have been no recourse for the workers.

Some years ago Greyhound Bus Lines made the statement that the human body begins to degenerate after the age of 35! They began retiring their drivers in their mid-50s. However, because of the laws against discrimination in aging, they lost their case when the Labor Department proved that they had superb drivers who were over the age of 60.

However, in another case, it was the government which contended that 60 was a magic age of physical dissolution, when the Federal Aviation Administration instituted mandatory retirement for commercial pilots at that age. As one pilot observed in a protest held in Washington, "One day you're 59 and you're up there flying, and the next day you're out."

The problem was studied by a panel of physicians for ten months. They concluded that there is "no special significance" to the age of 60 as a mandatory retirement standard. In fact, they strongly recommended that greater emphasis be placed on determining the ability of individual pilots to meet medical criteria for flying commercial jets, rather than on an arbitrary age. Sometime later I was reading a newspaper and came across an article that made me smile. It spoke of a man named Russell Green who had always had an interest in flying but just never could get around to it until later in life. He took his oral and flight tests with the FAA and passed. He now has behind him over 200 solo flights in gliders. He's 83 years of age!

This whole subject of retirement is but another example of how preposterous it is to attempt to put an entire generation into a neat package of predictability. Some of us want to retire and some of us already have, and many of us will be dragged screaming into this vague mixture of stereotypes, myths, dreams, fantasies, fears, anticipations, and sudden discoveries of new realities when we finally do surrender.

Whatever our choice, though, there is a real need to assess retirement in sober, unromantic terms if we are to make it a successful change in the patterns of our lives. It need not be a crisis, though it sometimes appears to be. We have been raised in the American work ethic and suddenly that commitment has been taken away from us— to be replaced, I hope, by something different, something new, and possibly something just as rewarding, if not more so. "You can retire," Maggie Kuhn says, "but you can't retire from life."

I roamed the shopping centers and the parking malls in Florida and Arizona and California and I spoke with men and women who had settled there—some with dreams, some with resignation, some with the anticipation of finally doing what they had wanted to do and had worked hard to achieve. Depending on the expectations and the acceptance of reality, these places are either anterooms to the grave or doorways to euphoria and castles in the air.

I met him while standing on line in a department store in Miami. His first words were, "Are you retired?" I answered that I was not, and we went out to a shopping mall coffee shop to talk. He had owned his own company, had sold it, and had just retired a few months before. The realities were beginning to settle in.

"When I gave up my office, I gave up my throne," he told me. He was not unusual. The feeling of having somewhere to go, something structured to do, was gone and the adjustment was taking place slowly but unmistakably. The office "perks" were still clearly recalled and "when I had to pay for the first tankful of gas, it nearly killed me!"

I wandered about for days, sitting on benches and talking to other retired people. Outside the shops the men waited, ready to discourse on businesses past and deals once consummated and work no longer theirs. There was talk of illnesses shared and sons (rarely daughters) who were doing well as doctors or lawyers back in New York or Los Angeles or Chicago.

In the supermarkets the *couples* shop together, rather than the women alone who did the marketing while the husband played king in the office. Retirement, for both men and women, is suddenly finding a new face around all the time. The person who showed up for dinner only occasionally is now always there at dinnertime—and at breakfast and lunch too! People who barely saw each other are now living together 24 hours a day. Too much spare time hangs heavily and too many retirees feel like displaced persons, seeing the world much differently than they had expected to see it; unprepared; certain that every minor ache is the first sign of disability or chronic disease. There is disenchantment, the pinch of inflation, the children who visit too seldom or who make their duty-bound annual visit around Christmas. Somehow, none of it was foreseen.

The "Paradise" of my father and others like him also carries with it exactly the same problems that he encountered in New York or that would confront him in Detroit or Omaha or Boston. In the retirement communities of the Sun Belt, I find that people carry guns on the seats of their cars and in their glove compartments. On my way to an interview in Florida, I turn on the radio and I hear a commercial recommending that I quickly purchase chemical mace! "Be careful of rip-offs if your car breaks down. Protect your family. It stuns with no ill effect for up to 15 minutes!"

In the local supermarket a small magazine, published for people who own condominiums, carries the headline, "Problems in Condos. Violence, Registering Pets, Cults and More." I feel that I am back in New York looking at a terrible local tabloid that uses scare headlines to boost circulation. Somehow reality has followed the retirees where it was not supposed to go. I don't know whether to laugh or find someone to whom I can read aloud when the stories tell of dead chickens being placed on a unit owner's doorstep. A Broward County Circuit Court transcript speaks of a couple who were sitting near their pool and got into an argument with two men who pulled down the bathing trunks of the husband and "proceeded to strike and punch the plaintiff into a state of senselessness."

A condominium association president is bitten in the leg by a cultist. An apartment owner threatens to kill the president of another association with his shotgun because he moved the man's bicycle from the common parking area. Dog excrement is thrown into the swimming pool from the balcony of a posh terrace in a high-rise building.

The condominiums of Florida, the cooperatives of Southern California, and the retirement homes in small villages of the Sun Belt have been painted as insulation from the day-to-day problems of the "outside world." We expect our retired lives to be free of care, empty of all worry, devoid of responsibility. They are, in fact, bubbling cauldrons that reflect the very life styles of the world we have just left, with the added complications of a major psychological and physical readjustment. The retirees who remain within the communities in which they've lived all their lives are often better able to accept the fact that the real world continues just as it has all along, in spite of their own change of life style.

I suppose it is my prerogative deliberately to paint a dark and brooding picture in order to make my point. Too much is expected with too little planning, and it is no different from the way in which we spend the rest of our lives—with denial of reality, lack of forethought, and a refusal to confront and accept changes and turning points as anything but a crisis. Are there happy retirees? Indeed there are, and almost all of them have met the two prime prerequisites for success in retirement:

> ◢ Sufficient financial planning to make life comfortable and moderately worry-free.
> ◢ Some planned continuation of interests, be it through new careers, volunteer work, or even fishing. Most have set some goal for themselves and *all* have accepted the fact that they cannot retire from life.

My brother-in-law, Murray, planned for his retirement from the day he started working. For him, the idea of leisure with enough income on which to live was the goal, his driving force, his ultimate achievement. He retired at 55 and moved to Florida, the very place that I so easily dismissed earlier in this chapter. He is doing exactly what he set out to do and he is one of the happiest people I know, with time to spend on investment detail, friends he knew back in the Northeast, and an absolute aversion to ever returning to the cold winters of New York.

Some hours ago I spent a wonderful morning interviewing two friends here on Fire Island, both of whom retired a few years ago, though not at exactly the same time. "It was deliberate," Tom says. "There is an adjustment period to retirement, being home all the time with someone who has been a 'weekend spouse' all these years. So I retired first and Norma joined me two years later."

Both Tom and Norma are two of the most contented retirees I've ever met. He is an ex-NBC executive and lawyer and he has used his retirement to achieve all the travel plans he's ever dreamed of, from Egypt to the Galapagos Islands off Ecuador; to engage in astronomy, fishing, sailing, and so many other activities that we find it difficult to keep track of his current interests. "I also like to putter," he explains. "But," he continues, "the key is to retire on your own terms if you can. All the unsuccessful retirements I saw at NBC were because of two things—financial problems or not knowing what to do with all that time for all those days. The happiest retirement party I ever saw at the network was for a long-time researcher who had planned *15 years* for just that moment. He showed pictures of the farm he had bought, spoke of what he was going to do with it, and probably had a better time at that party than anyone else!"

Norma had been the administrative manager for a large law firm and now she is more active than ever in the politics of our island. She served first as mayor of our village and was one of the best administrators we've ever had. She is now in her first term as president of the Fire Island Association, an active group of citizens interested in preserving this most fragile barrier reef and protecting it against overdevelopment and the incursions of urban civilization. "You have to keep busy," she agrees. "Every morning, you wake up with a mental list of what you are going to get done—and it somehow never gets done!"

My friend Dee, who wrote so eloquently about the "empty nest" earlier in this book, has just sent a letter that tells me he is retiring as an executive of the Coca-Cola Company at the age of 55, so that he can go back to school to get his master's degree! Still another friend, retired for about two years, told me, "I'm so busy, I'm surprised that I had time for *work* all those years!"

"Are there happy retirees?" Maggie Kuhn answers, "Yes, I think there are. First of all, they have an income that is sufficient to offset the ravages of inflation. Also, they've had enough in their own past experience to enable them to define their goals and start again. Some people see old age as an extension of what they have been doing before, rather than a freedom, a new beginning for new roles, and a liberated kind of spirit of adventure and risk taking. It's an opportunity to rebuild and to try something entirely new."

When we interview retirees about their past, they generally say that the most important thing the job brought them, next to the income, was the work itself, the feeling of being useful, and the activity that took place around them for at least eight hours a day. For some executives bordering on the workaholic, the *only* thing that satisfied them was their involvement with work—up to 16 hours each and every day, weekends included.

When people do retire, the Harris study found, most do not want to be excluded from the world around them, nor limited to communities of other people of their own age. Of even more interest are the figures dealing with what retired people feel are the most important steps to take in preparing for our later years:

📖 88 percent consider it very important to have medical care available.
📖 81 percent, to prepare a will.
📖 80 percent, to build up savings.
📖 80 percent, to learn about and investigate pensions and Social Security benefits.
📖 70 percent, to buy one's own home.
📖 64 percent, to develop leisure-time activities.
📖 50 percent, to decide whether to move or continue to live in the same area.
📖 31 percent, to plan a new part-time or full-time job.

Notice, if you will, the preoccupation with finances. The major regrets for already retired people lie mainly in this area and many wish that they had planned their careers differently in order to guarantee greater security. Unfortunately, this is an area in which most of us do not have total control, but awareness and planning are at least the first small steps.

There are hundreds of books, pamphlets, and articles about retirement and if we were to condense all the good advice, it boils down simply to this: get started now in your planning. If you are so driven by your work that you have developed no outside interests at all, now might be a good time to take stock. My friend Larry retired from the Suffolk County police force at the age of 42. His hobby of clockmaking and watch repair turned into a lucrative business in Florida. It might be well for *you* to make a list of all the things that have interested you these 40 or 50 or 60 years, aside from the work world.

Look carefully at what your retirement budget is going to be and see if you can live on it for a month, taking into consideration the inflationary rate, your investments, and the possibility of some outside income from additional work.

I must assume that you and your spouse (if there is one) are very compatible. Don't discount the potential conflicts and readjustments when the retiree suddenly appears permanently in someone else's "space."

Dr. Erdman Palmore, professor of medical sociology at the Center for the Study of Aging and Development at Duke University, even recommends that you take a month off for a "trial retirement" in order to learn to develop new routines and work out the new territorial claims with your spouse.

If you're working at a large corporation, you may find that counseling is available for preretirement employees, not only in financial matters but also in planning medical coverage and handling the social and emotional problems that may arise. Some community colleges and schools of continuing education also are offering retirement counseling programs.

One of the best series of preretirement and retirement pamphlets is published by the American Association of Retired Persons (1909 K Street N.W., Washington, DC 20049) and is available for a small annual membership fee. They cover *Finance, Income Taxes, Tips on Retirement, Health and Insurance Programs, Generic Prescription Drugs, Housing, Age Discrimination, Crime Prevention, Community Service, Widowhood, Nutrition,* and much, much more. You may not read all of them, but they'll start you thinking about all the areas that may become more important to you in the coming years. They may, indeed, help avoid what sociologists sometimes call "retirement shock."

Maggie Kuhn is right. You do not retire from living, from being a consumer. As she says, however black the humor, "You use and consume products right through rigor mortis! You even are a consumer in the way you're interred, cremated, or buried at sea, a fancy funeral that gets the undertaker richer. We are all consumers." We cannot retire from the world, from being responsible citizens, from fighting for what we think is right. Our talents need not wither because of still another change in this ever-changing life of ours.

I look at where I am now, in my late 50s, and I cannot answer the question of whether or not I will retire. Will I do all the things for which I've made lists all these years? I have never visited the Statue of Liberty, I am ashamed to admit, though it lies at the door of my city. There has been no time to tie up the grapes in the arbor outside, no time to go up to the Bronx Zoo to see the 150-pound baby elephant just born there, no time to read some of the new books that pass by me in a frenzy of publishing mania, nor to reread some of my old favorites like *Catcher in the Rye*.

Somehow, though I can fully empathize with those of my brothers and sisters who *do* want to retire, I feel at this point in my life that, just like my friend Norma, I will continue to make lists that I cannot ever get to, jobs that I will never accomplish. I cannot see the end of my filmmaking, for I hope that I shall become better as I age. I have books scheduled in my head for 50 years to come. I would like to do a novel, but I am still slightly wary of the challenge. Possibly I am too young to attempt it yet!

My father, whose seed was responsible in part for creating my own neurotic, hypertensive personality, is beginning to threaten. Paradise is not only lost—it was never there to begin with. He wants to come back to New York, weather, problems, and all. He admits, in his weaker moments, that it might not work, but he continues to threaten and I encourage him. If he wants to return, I will do all I can to make it easier. For now—and I do not know how I will feel in 20 years—he is right. It is better here, if that is what he thinks.

In all the weeks and months of speaking to retired people about this book, I find that my father is not alone, not by any means. My friend and accountant, Dave Ribet, tells of a telephone call that he received from a friend who had retired to Florida. Exasperated, frustrated, irritated, the man exploded on the telephone with, "Good God, Dave! How many sprinklers can I fix? How many rounds of golf can I play? How many times can I have coffee with the boys? I must come back to New York and have some *aggravation!*"

I understand. I do understand. At least for now.

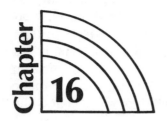

# The Case of the
# Incredible Shrinking Dollar

*Youth is the time of getting, middle age of improving, and old age of spending.*

> Anne Bradstreet
> *(17th century):*
> Thirty-Three Meditations

A short time ago, on a film trip through California, our crew stopped for a quick, indescribably bad airport lunch while waiting for a connecting plane. Our assistant cameraman, about 30 years old, ordered his two hamburgers, french-fried potatoes, chocolate malted, and a dessert of fresh, out-of-season strawberries priced at around $3.50 for six plump, artificially grown fruit. Since he was obviously a fast-food aficionado, he devoured the first part of his lunch with gusto and then pulled the small bowl of strawberries toward him.

Tenderly, he lifted one red berry to his lips, took a single small bite, put it back in the bowl, and pushed the remainder away, untouched, in a single gesture of indifference. Curious, I asked him if they were spoiled or possibly tasteless. "Oh no," he answered. "That's all I really wanted." Our cameraman, Joe Longo, sensing my dismay at the waste, looked at me with a twinkle in his eye and silently mouthed the word, "Spoiled!" Being close to my age, Joe obviously understood exactly what was going through my head.

I am a child of the Depression, and I have never been able to shake completely the feelings that come with the memories of that distant time in our history. It is true that our family kept most of the anguish and despair from my brother and me. It is also true that later years more than made up for that struggle through the uniquely American opportunity that allowed an immigrant family to move into the middle class. As a child I was only too aware that the times were formidable. My father had to work too many hours. The urban reflections of the dust bowl and its gaunt, hungry farmers were seen in the faces of our city's apple sellers. I can still see my father's fearful expression when he ran from the house one morning to join the growing line at the shuttered neighborhood bank where a lifetime of savings had suddenly been sealed behind closed doors. I remember entire families being thrust out into the street, their furniture, their clothing, and their pathetically few other possessions piled on the sidewalk, as distraught mothers tried to comfort their bewildered children.

I cannot tolerate waste. Even the lettuce or parsley used as a garnish in most of America's restaurants, and left on the plate by almost all diners, to be thrown out, is a sin to me. I envision the farmer who grew the crop having nightmares as he contemplates the results of his efforts ending up as grist for a giant sanitation truck. So, in spite of the fact that I have joined the ranks of one of the most affluent of groups in American history, the insecurities of those early times remain with me, and I am convinced that everything in life is temporary. I wait, appearing to be secure, for the sword of Damocles to fall and take it all away. My background asserts itself only too strongly in my reaction to watching the waste of a bowl of strawberries. And it is something our children and our children's children will never understand.

It stands to reason, then, that someone who is like me—I assume that there are others who feel exactly the same way—would be concerned and terribly uneasy over the headlines that greet one each morning in the newspapers and magazines. If, as I stated in the previous chapter, my future as an older American is very much related to the financial structure that I am building as a middle-aged person, my apprehensions are understandable. For those of us in these middle years, a promise is being threatened. We are being told that Social Security is in dire trouble. We are being told that we, who are next in line to depend upon this enlightened system of financial insurance, will probably find that the cupboard is bare!

For me, as for millions of others who are middle-aged, Social

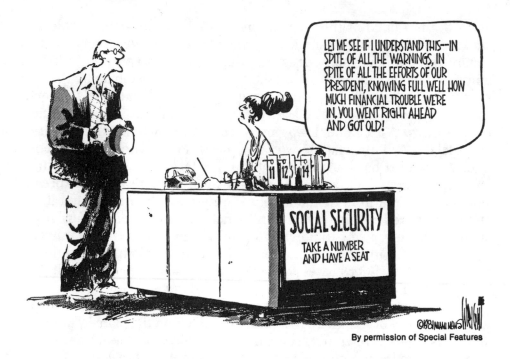

By permission of Special Features

Security is an integral part of a plan that includes private pension plans or an IRA (Individual Retirement Account) plus some small investments and insurance. If you take away any part of it, our entire financial structure suffers. It is difficult to plan the next 20 years or more without being constantly reminded of an impending catastrophe. And, oh, how prevalent those reminders are!

*Newsweek* magazine prints a cover story, "Can You Afford to Retire?" Other headlines compete for my attention, many of them on the very first page of the newspapers:

> Turmoil in Pension Plans
> The Crisis (sic!) in Social Security
> Retiring at Age 65 a Receding Goal
> Elderly Get Grim News for Future

To top it all off, an administration that seems to be totally insensitive to the needs, the fears, and the aspirations of so many millions of us takes office in Washington. A smiling President makes a TV address to the nation (July 27, 1981) and states that "I will not stand by and see those of you who are dependent upon Social Security deprived of your benefits. I make that pledge to you as your President. You have no reason to be frightened." And he continued to smile. Of course, only two days later, a White House spokesman stated that the President's pledge did *not* apply to those who were receiving the minimum benefit. As the scare stories continued to be published, I began to think that the smiling President was actually laughing at us, and it began to get much worse.

The Treasury Secretary was asked at a meeting of New York financial writers just how he thought Social Security will be funded 50 years from now, and he replied, "I don't know. I'll be dead by then." As my grandmother used to say, "With friends like that, you don't need enemies!"

What are we being told? What, indeed, are the reasons for the warnings, the scare stories, the words about "nothing to fear" while at the same time other words threaten the structure of an entire social system? The Social Security Act, signed by Pres. Franklin Delano Roosevelt in 1935, is one of the most outstanding pieces of social legislation in this century, providing dignity and a measure of security for more than 36 million working people. The statistics upon which it was based were viable and very practical.

For every 35 workers there was only one retiree, and the surplus grew large enough to expand the system to include additional trust funds for disability insurance, dependents and survivors, Medicare, and supplementary medical insurance. It was successful beyond the wildest dreams of Roosevelt and the Congress of 1935. It dramatically reduced the number of elderly poor to just about 15 percent as we enter this decade. It has provided a secure base for future financial planning for people in middle age, since it also incorporates cost-of-living increases at prescribed intervals. And now, we are being told, it has collided head-on with some sobering demographics.

They tell us that when it all began, 35 working people supported a single pensioner, and for the first 12 years or so, each worker was taxed only 1 percent on a maximum ceiling of $3,000, or $30 per year—small even by post-Depression standards. As people began to live longer and retire earlier, the ratio plummeted and the burden was forced upon fewer and fewer workers. Today only 3 workers support the payments for each retiree, and the tax is approaching 7.05 percent in 1985, applied to earnings up to $43,500, for a maximum of $3,066 per year. In 1990 the rate will rise to 7.65 percent and the base will jump to $66,900 a year, for a maximum tax of $5,117.

The voices of Washington also tell us that the economy has not helped matters. High unemployment has reduced the number of people paying taxes into the trust fund, while the double-digit inflation rate has increased the cost of benefits to retirees. Over the next five years, we are told, the Social Security system faces a shortage of between 10 billion and 100 billion dollars (depending upon whose figures you use), and a still more serious crisis will occur in about 25 to 30 years when the "baby boom" workers reach maturity and begin to retire. So much has been written about this "crisis," and the voices of doom have been so loud and persistent, that most people at age 30 do not believe they will ever see one cent of their Social Security taxes returned to them when they reach retirement age—whether it be an early 50 or a later 70.

It is no accident that I have used the words, "What are we being told?" for the more I watch the scenario unfold, the more I suspect we are being made the victims for a host of *other* governmental problems with the economy.

I am no longer alone in my cynicism, and the voices of reason and advocacy are beginning to be heard. At a small gathering of friends this past summer, I spoke at length with Congresswoman Geraldine Ferraro (D-Queens), a member of the Select Committee on Aging in the House of Representatives. We spoke of the financial *Titanic* being predicted by the administration whenever the subject of Social Security arose. Finally, she laughed, and said, "You don't believe everything they tell you, I hope?" And she suggested that I contact Robert M. Ball. It was a name I had heard before.

Robert M. Ball served as Commissioner of Social Security under three administrations in Washington, dating back to 1962, then became a consultant in 1973. He is currently the Chairman of the Advisory Committee of the "Save Our Social Security" (SOS) Coalition, made up of over 90 organizations with a combined membership of about 40 million adults. Indeed, I am not alone, for the coalition includes labor unions, senior citizen groups, groups that represent the disabled, the major church groups, and social welfare groups. Though Bob Ball and the coalition are aware that the Social Security system will need additional income over these next few years, he says rather strongly that

".. . this can and should be done without further reducing Social Security benefits for those now receiving them and without reducing promised protection for those now contributing to the program."

Why this strange dichotomy, this strong difference of opinion between the administration doomsayers and people like Bob Ball, U.S. Representatives Claude Pepper and Geraldine Ferraro, and a growing number of members of Congress who sit on both sides of the aisle— not to mention the doubters like you and me? Why the diametrically opposed projections, now being called by more and more economists a "spurious bankruptcy" issue?

Simply put, the administration, in projecting its original economic program, projected the best performance for the economy and the "supply-side" theory—more productivity, greater employment, and a lowering of the interest rates and inflation. When the figures for Social Security and other social programs were projected, the "worst case" assumptions were used. Bob Ball, in testimony prepared for the Committee of the Budget, House of Representatives (October 1981), put it, ".. . under the 'worst case' assumptions, which the Administration wants to use for Social Security purposes but no other, there could be difficulty as early as 1984 or 1985. These assumptions include double-digit inflation through 1984, no real wage increases over the next five years, and unemployment reaching nearly 10 percent by 1983. Now there is a possibility that economic conditions might be this bad, and the Social Security system does not need to be protected against such a possibility."

He agrees that there are now 3.2 people working for each retired person, but he strongly states that the projection of only 2 workers for each retired person in the year 2020 is not a fact, but an assumption. "More older people are likely to be working then, and also more women," he stated in an interview. "There will be fewer young people for the working population to support. Fertility rates may change, and so may immigration policy and productivity, all of which affect the picture. I refuse to accept that it's necessary to cut benefits now because this future problem is more or less inevitable."

There are many solutions for both the short term and the long term, and considering the political implications of the changes that have been suggested, there is a good chance that some way will be found to keep the trust fund alive and well. In the first place, in spite of what the administration would like us to believe, it is *not* the public— us and our younger colleagues—who would rebel against the rising taxes needed to keep the Social Security system solvent. The Harris study found that an overwhelming majority of the general public—young *and* old—feel that the government should help support older people with taxes collected from everyone. As a matter of fact, those under 65 were even stronger in their feelings than those over 65! Ninety-seven percent agreed that "as the cost of living increases, Social Security payments to retired people should also increase."

Bob Ball adds, "It is worth noting, in any event, that an 8½ percent rate is not an overwhelming burden, *even today*. German workers already pay 8 percent for old-age, survivors' and disability insurance protection and, in addition, the general revenues of the German government pay for 19 percent of the cost of the system."

So the single area of the tax increase is not the most objectionable one to the general public. It is (again) the corporations, the business community, looking for ways to cut their expenses, which object. As worker contributions rise, so do the amounts paid by the company—multiplied sometimes by thousands of employees. And suggestions to bolster Social Security by adding to the fund with general revenues, as in the German system, have also elicited loud screams of pain from the business community, which would have to bear the brunt of the burden.

There are, indeed, a hundred solutions that have been offered, many of them quite viable and practical for the long run as well as the short term. There have been suggestions to raise the retirement age to 68 by gradually moving it up month by month until the year 2000. Anyone retiring before that age would be severely penalized by reduced income. Unfortunately, there are some very good arguments *against* this seemingly simple plan: some people are forced to retire because of ill health or "burn-out" on the job—and it would be wonderful if we could first eliminate age-discrimination on all levels of the corporate world before we decided to keep our employees there three years longer.

Some options include eliminating the ceiling on additional earnings for retirees on Social Security; calculating the amount of retirement pay on actual earnings; enacting a national sales tax; phasing out student benefits; interfund borrowing from areas such as hospital insurance or from the general fund at market interest rates; changing the calculation of the inflation rate and cost-of-living increases; and broadening Social Security through universal coverage of *all* employees, both in the private sector and in the government. The latter suggestion would, no doubt, raise a storm that would make the corporate complaints seem a whisper by comparison! Federal employees, for example, can take early retirement at age 55 with full benefits, and their cost-of-living increases are figured twice a year.

But I have saved the best for last, and it is the single most important reason that I have the optimism to even suggest that something will be done to guarantee that Social Security will be around for a long time. In the political arena, we middle-aged people and our elderly brothers and sisters represent the most awesome, single-issue block of voters in the country today. Each of us is affected by every suggestion, every option, and every word spoken by the administration and in Congress on the subject of Social Security and our financial futures. The first move of the executive branch was to stop the payments of the minimum amount ($122) to a wide range of needy recipients. It was not too long afterward that Congress acted and the headline in the *New York Times* (October 16, 1981) read: "Senate, 95-0, Acts to Save Solvency of Social Security," including a return to the base benefit.

The issue is a volatile one, and the battle will continue, and the skirmishes will echo through the country long after this book has gone to press. I suggest that we all step back and take a good hard look before we accept the scare stories and the headlines that portend a quicksand of disaster. *We,* the middle-aged and the elderly, refuse to carry more than our share of the drastic cutbacks and broken promises, while budgets are increased astronomically for cruise missiles, B-1 bombers, and neutron weapons; while the sugar and tobacco lobbies manage to keep their own support systems afloat in Congress; and while the oil companies are targeted for special tax relief.

I have said that I am, by nature, suspicious and somewhat of a cynic, especially when it comes to what we are told "is good for you." I have worked, as you may have done, hard and long to make my way in this world. As a former Depression kid, I carry with me the memories of the human problems that led to our great social programs—especially a Social Security system that has been called "America's most civilized project." I also retain my faith in the thinking and the legislative skills of a group of brilliant, enlightened, and farseeing people who understood what it meant for millions to face a future of broken dreams.

Claude Pepper wrote, "Social Security is your rightful return on a lifelong investment in hard work" and Bob Ball adds, ". . . it is much more than an antipoverty program. Social Security is the base on which just about everyone in the United States builds protection against the loss of earned income because of retirement in old age, total disability, and death. Every private pension plan in the United States is based on the assumption that the pensioner will also receive a Social Security benefit, and individuals who are saving on their own, count on Social Security as a base for their efforts."

It is no accident, then, that the architects of Social Security created a payroll tax as the means of funding the system. Once we have contributed, it is then our *right* to claim the benefits when we retire, and we must be terribly vigilant to see that the government's part of the bargain is kept. There has been no charity involved, no paternalistic funding by our companies or by the government. *We* have paid the taxes for all these years. *We* are entitled to the benefits, and with all the cries of "crisis" in the hallowed halls of the executive branch, I have no doubt that our politically sensitive legislators will find a solution.

Our President has a penchant for quoting Franklin Delano Roosevelt. It might be enlightening for him and for the members of his economic staff and the elected members of Congress to look carefully at the statement that FDR made after Social Security had been signed into law. With regard to the tax structure of the system, he said, "Those taxes were never a problem of economics. They are *political* all the way through. We put those payroll contributions there so as to give the contributors a legal, moral, and political right to collect their pensions. With those taxes in there, *no damn politician can ever scrap my Social Security program!*"

Those of us of middle age and older are watching carefully to see if FDR will be heard throughout the land.

# Part IV
# New Beginnings,
# New Horizons

On a barrier island there are familiar and very special harbingers of autumn. Early this morning, as I watched the ocean curl toward the beach, the small yellow school bus made its way slowly over the sand for the first time. The driver and I waved to each other. I looked toward the whitecaps to see if I might detect the first run of autumn bluefish in the surf.

The summer renters have departed, hauling their packed city belongings atop the little wagons down to the ferry dock, reminding me of Tevye in *Fiddler on the Roof* as he and his family left Anatevka, their household goods piled high on a rickety cart. Soon the ducks will form their fluttering lines as they head south. The monarch butterflies will make their annual migration, to fill the walks with orange-black wings. The purple beach plums hang heavy on the scraggly bushes near the sand dunes, and the August noises have given way to the insistent sounds of the September crickets and click-beetles. It has become so very quiet and peaceful again.

I have passed my 58th birthday in the writing of this book, and I have had almost a year to think about the change in life style that I chose for myself during just such a September of reflection, self-evaluation, and contemplation. I have stated before that the very idea of change is usually quite difficult for me: Mental turmoil accompanies even the slightest digression from the status quo. If I cannot bear to see the furniture moved within a room, imagine my reaction to the rearrangement of my whole life style!

It has been a year of change and the result has been a good one, though not without readjustments, which I shall discuss more fully in the chapter that follows. But perhaps more important than my personal traumas or exhilaration has been the discovery that I am not alone in changing the direction of my life. There are literally millions of people of our generations who are taking stock: reevaluating their personal and business lives: finding new freedoms, new interests, new doors to open. If we were not so damned invisible, the world would soon be aware that we are very much like the ocean that roars and churns not far from where I write—constantly changing; first roiling, then placid; searching its way onto the beach, withdrawing, then moving in again; constantly probing and resculpting the earth beneath it. I, who protest so much that I cannot tolerate change, find that very change exciting, both in my piece of ocean and in my life.

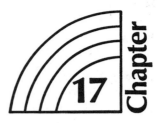

# What Do You Want to Be When You Grow Up?

> *For each age is a dream that is dying, Or one that is coming to birth.*
>
> *Arthur O'Shaughnessy:*
> Ode

The luncheon had already been in progress for over an hour and, for my part, I could have stayed in the restaurant the remainder of the afternoon. My companion, who had just turned 50, was fascinating, easy to talk with, and filled with an enthusiasm and a life force that characterize so many of my contemporaries. We moved from subject to subject, leaning forward in our involvement, paying little attention to the captain and the waiters, finding much to agree on, laughing, probing. "Who are we?" he asked, rhetorically. We agreed that we were very special generations and he continued, ticking off his points on his fingers.

"We lived through the '30s and we were seared by the Depression. We lived through the '40s and we were scarred by the war. We lived through the '50s and we learned to keep our mouths shut and get along in the world. In the '60s—which we also lived through—we found that the flower children were successful at doing their own thing. In 171 the '70s we saw that the kids of the '60s might have been saying something to *us*, and it began to have relevancy in our own changes. We go into the '80s asking, 'How about me?' "

I met Dr. James Gallagher after reading an article about him in the business section of the *New York Times*. He is chairman of a group called Career Management Associates, and he and his staff devote their time to "outplacement," the counseling of middle-aged executives who have been "separated"—a contemporary word to soften the real meaning: *fired*. They are people who have devoted most of their lives to the corporation, and being fired in their late 40s or 50s is possibly one of the most shattering experiences that can occur in their adult lives. Dr. Gallagher equates it with the death of a family member, a serious injury, or being sent to jail for a felony.

What struck me most, however, was his attitude, his optimism, and, most of all, his conclusion that most fired executives, properly counseled, can end up with even better-paying jobs, usually in a field other than the one to which they have devoted so much of their working lives.

I was curious. Through my years in dealing with major corporations and producing their films, I had seen many executives either fired after the age of 50 or moved "sideways" into a job with no future. Some of these people were clients with whom I had developed a long and close relationship and I suffered right along with them. Some were forced to take early retirement; others were the victims of cost-cutting after disappointing annual profit projections. Several of my closest friends were passed over for a vice-presidency because they were too close to retirement and, after 30 to 40 years with the company, they watched silently as a replacement was brought in from the outside to become their superior. For me, all of it was tied together—the deliberate insulation of the corporation from humanity has been evident all through my career, and the age-discrimination in the decisions only too obvious. The irony, of course, is that many of those decisions to fire a long-time employee are being made by people of *our own age,* unaware that they may well be next.

So I spoke at length to Dr. Gallagher, for I felt that if I could understand what happens during a middle-age termination, and if Dr. Gallagher could be so positive about such severe dislocations, what would his attitude be toward those of us who *voluntarily* decide to change our life styles and those of us who choose to remain active in the corporate world past the age of "normal" retirement—either with the companies with which we've spent 30 or more years, or in a major shift to another field of endeavor?

The long luncheon and several clarifying telephone calls followed and, through it all, what fascinated me most was that *not once* in our discussions did the word "crisis" ever rear its ugly snout!

"We live under a set of assumptions that make life liveable—that the power will go on when we switch on the light, that the buses will run." He went on, enthusiastically. "And we were given other assumptions, were we not? Start at the bottom. Keep your nose clean. Work hard. You will be successful. But those assumptions—as all others--do not take into account *change.*" (There was that word again.) He leaned forward. "Look, if we've lived on this planet for 50 years or more, we've had to accommodate change—the aerospace revolution, the cold war, inflation, even the advent of television. We've absorbed them all into our family life, in society, education and in government. Why not in our careers?"

He laughed. "I remember all my young life I lived under the assumption that FDR would always be President. I was led to assume that the presidency was a stable reference in my life. I was born a Roman Catholic. I was led to assume that, if I went to Communion for the first Friday of nine consecutive months, I would go to Heaven. Well, they've changed the rules! The mass is no longer in Latin. I can eat meat on Friday. I don't have to fast before Communion; I can have water or coffee first. *The constant is change!*"

And thus our assumption is that if we work hard and we stay with the corporation, always trustworthy, loyal, thrifty, clean, and brave, we will be rewarded. But one day, to our regret, that assumption is blasted. I have seen the looks on the faces of the terminated middle-aged executives who come to Dr. Gallagher's office. It is not a pleasant experience.

According to Jim Gallagher, the fired employee goes through two major stages. The first one begins with disbelief: "This really isn't happening to me." This is followed by anger—threatening to "knock somebody's block off" or burying it deeply within, possibly to surface at the wrong time in a subsequent job interview, only to hurt the candidate's chances. Then comes a period of bargaining—trying to find a way to save the job, threatening to see the president, asking for time to look around for a transfer within the corporation. But bargaining is futile.

Dr. Gallagher illustrates the final point in the first stage, bargaining, with an anecdote from Dr. Elisabeth Kübler-Ross's work with hospital patients who were terminally ill. One woman bargained with her doctor to keep her well enough to attend the wedding of her oldest son, even though she could not survive her advanced cancer. Through the doctor's skill, her persistence, and a great deal of luck, she went to the wedding. When she returned to the hospital after the ceremony and reception, she met the doctor, smiled, and greeted him with, "Don't forget, doctor, I have another son!"

During the second stage of the termination period, depression replaces the initial shock, followed by gradual acceptance of the situation and the building of hope through sheer determination. It is during this period that the individual is forced to review his total past experience and to prepare for a job search, develop his strategy, collect names, and produce an effective résumé. The move then is into the positive activity of a job search. The success rate, sometimes after another small dip into depression—usually about the sixth week—is amazingly good. Through intensive counseling, people are induced to search deeply, and many a new job reflects a talent in an area never even thought of before!

Dr. Gallagher's statistics are interesting, considering the fact that the trauma of being fired during middle age seems so hopeless and irreparable. Over the years, for those who have been professionally counseled by Dr. Gallagher's organization and others like it:

> It took, on the average, about one week of job search for each $2,000 of annual salary before the individual was placed.
> About 60 percent of the executives and managers who received outplacement guidance came through with new jobs within 20 weeks.
> *About 85 percent found jobs at a higher salary than they had received before they were fired.*
> About 2 percent thought it was about time to start their own businesses.

Keep in mind that these are figures for people who had no choice in the matter. Why, then, do we hesitate to make a move from an unrewarding situation when the decision is totally ours? Generally, because we have been taught to think that we are too old to start again.

As we grow older, we are conditioned to deny our own worth and the intrinsic values and attributes that we bring to our society, if only through our greater experience. The virulence of age-discrimination in our culture begins to affect even those of us who should know better, when we hear ourselves declaring, "We have to make way for young ideas and young blood." We accept too quickly the words of the chairman of the board who fires two top officers in their 70s because they are "stagnating" and are "not attuned to the times." The same chief executive officer was quoted in the *Wall Street Journal* as saying that the company needed "younger, more aggressive leaders" while being totally insensitive to his own age of 68! He is, as much as any of us, a victim of the youth culture in America.

The assumptions that Dr. Gallagher spoke of rule our lives and our attitudes about ourselves. We assume that we must live up to the expectations of others, that we must bow to the conventional ideas and criteria of our society. As Gay Gaer Luce says in her book, *Your Second Life*, "Our culture teaches us many ways to be unhealthy. . . . We are taught in first grade to stop feeling who we are ('You can stand in the closet if you're going to cry') and to give up our lives for good grades, reputation, and, later, money."

Is it any wonder that we begin to dislike ourselves and to agree with the myths about aging; to doubt our abilities; to assume that a traumatic change in middle life does irreparable damage to our dignity and our life style? Is it any wonder that a *voluntary* change of career at age 50 or later is greeted with "You must have guts!" It is another important area in our lives where the myths become self-perpetuating, and our assumptions begin to rule our behavior, what we think, what we say, what we write.

Our assumptions make us believe, for example, that *all* middle-aged people are heterosexual, yet many are lesbians, gay men, or bisexuals. Our assumptions about aging are such that we—the people in midlife—believe that our talents decrease as the years go by. Thus, in this very morning's newspaper, there is a review of a concert by Frank Sinatra that reads, in part, ". . . but for a man of 65, his technique is remarkable." Angrily I read on, and it was the next part of the review that showed the adulation the writer felt, and I wondered why Sinatra's age had to be mentioned at all: "In fact, every time this writer has heard him in recent years, his voice has seemed more secure and wider in range both for dynamics and pitch." Why is he surprised?

We tend to focus on the brilliant and powerful personalities in show business, in the corporate world, and in government to find the people who we think are *exceptions* to the rule of retirement at a specific age. Scientists and engineers do their most celebrated work late in their 60s and 70s. Writers, artists, doctors, lawyers, and professors remain active into their 80s and experience some of their best years after the onset of middle age.

When I first began to collect the vast profusion of materials that now fill my office, closets, and file cabinets, I thought I might compile a listing that would clearly show how vital we all are. Unfortunately, I discovered two things at about the same time:

    📖 The "exceptions" to the rule—the woman sports editor at age 92, the 82-year-old preacher, the 90-year-old psychiatrist, the 72-year-old architect—all smacked of tokenism, exactly the kind of publicity that perpetuates the myth that these people *are* exceptions.

    📖 In fact, people such as I've mentioned above are more the *rule* than the exception. Had I begun such a list, it would have filled the space of ten bookshelves, set in type much smaller than this!

Not only is the President of the United States a prime example of successful career change in later years, but I look at the list of directors in a company in which I hold stock. The eight men are all over 54 and the eldest is 86. (The one woman director has modestly withheld her age from the annual report.)

The list of "who's who" in the corporate world, those who are "making way for younger blood," includes executives of some of the largest and most successful multinational corporations in the country. In the fields of publishing, communications, real estate, investment and finance, retailing, engineering, and aerospace, it carries so many chief executives who are over 70 that it must be embarrassing when they realize the extent to which they are marketing to the youth culture! Nor are they paying much heed to a statement made some time ago by Arjay Miller, former president of the Ford Motor Company, who was quoted as saying, "I don't think anyone over 70 should be chief executive of a large corporation. It helps the morale of a corporation to have turnover at the top; there are a lot of young bucks waiting to be chief."

In the sciences, in politics, in business, as well as in the arts, seldom are noteworthy achievements produced by people under 40, and many—if not most—take place from age 50 to well into the 80s. It is the *30-year-old* genius who is the exception, not the middle-aged achiever or the career changer.

What about the rest of us? What about those of us in middle age who do not hold the office of chief executive, either in the White House or in the board room of General Dynamics or the Columbia Broadcasting System? What about those of us who have never become even middle-level executives but have worked in the average office all our lives? What about those of us in our own businesses, in the retail world, in retirement, or in any career that suddenly seems to be giving less and less joy and rewards?

A report by the National Committee on Careers for Older Americans (*Older Americans: an Untapped Resource*. Academy for Educational Development, Inc., Washington, D.C., 1979) succinctly gives the all-too-common response of so many of us who have entered middle age: "Tragically, the other side of the coin is also commonplace. For whatever personal reasons, many highly trained and talented older people succumb to the depressing expectation that they should withdraw from life. . . . Sometimes these people are subject to their own or others' mistaken notion that their continued presence impedes the progress of younger people when, in fact, it is the younger people who benefit most by their continued leadership and example."

Let me set at least a part of the record straight. During World War II a great many older workers, including women who had not worked steadily since their teens, were employed in the defense industries while many of us marched off to Europe and the South Pacific. Studies of that era found that older workers had greater stability on the job, fewer accidents, and less time lost from work than did younger employees. More important, perhaps, is the fact that studies by the Department of Labor and the National Council on Aging concluded that older workers are able to produce work that is qualitatively and quantitatively *equal or superior to* that of the younger workers.

Older workers report more job satisfaction and less job-related stress than do younger employees. We are less likely to be absent, especially on the days when auto assembly lines turn out most of their "lemons"—Mondays and Fridays. The record shows, too, that we require less supervision, and that we have steadier work habits and a greater sense of responsibility and loyalty toward our jobs and our employers. Moreover, the reports indicate that we are less distracted by outside interests and influences, that we have fewer domestic troubles, and that we have higher levels of concentration than our young co-workers.

A few years ago I was hired to produce a film on the subject of "quality," and the sponsor of the project was one of the largest automobile manufacturers in the world. Armed with my questions, my camera crew, and my indomitable sense of optimism, I traveled to the assembly plant and, over the noise, clatter, and pounding—all the while dodging the slowly moving chasses—I tried to interview the workers about their feelings on "quality." My optimism soon vanished as the workers—particularly the *young ones*—met my questions with laughter, disbelief, and a series of unprintable responses for a film that would be shown to the general public.

"What would you do," I asked a young foreman, "if the people down the line forgot to punch the holes in which you put your grill-work?"

"We'd let it go by. If they don't do their job, we can't stop the line to do ours, can we?"

Another young man laughed and shouted loudly above the din, "Quality? Crap. I just want to finish this job this summer and get back to school!"

I came out of the project chastened, disturbed, and feeling much less naive. The older workers, either through being resigned, caring more, or carrying with them a stronger work ethic, were the ones who finally gave me the story I was looking for. I drive a 16-year-old car and I dread the day that I will have to replace it, for I will have to insist on an automobile made only by older workers!

How ironic! A culture of youth still persists in a society that has changed so much and is changing still. Billions of dollars have been thrown into the fight to improve nutrition, to increase the level of our medical care so that we can live longer, to increase our life span to the point where we are the fastest-growing segment of the entire population. In addition, our own attitudes are changing, making us *want* to continue to pursue active lives, unwilling to sit out our middle years and our retirement and possessing a greater range of skills and talent than ever before seen in an older population. How incomprehensible, then, that at this moment in time we are prone to aggravate this incredible waste of resources by demanding early retirement from the work force; that we exert subtle pressures to make way for the young; that we try every means to make millions of our population invisible and totally valueless! This ageism filters down even to the lowest economic levels. There has been a recent suggestion that the minimum-wage structure be eliminated for the teen-age group, something that would create still more firing of older workers. I note with amusement that it is being called "the great McDonald's giveaway."

Interestingly enough, both the assumptions and the rules are changing. The financial stress of double-digit inflation has made many of us determined to stay in the workplace or change our careers at mid-life. In addition, there is a growing awareness of just who we are, of our attributes and our power; a recognition of what has been a myth of middle age. I observe, as I see my peers, that there is a burgeoning sense of "self," that we are becoming cognizant of the fact that we can control much of the change that takes place throughout our adult lives.

Too often in our lives we are driven to change or to take risks only by pain. Jim Gallagher believes that the forces that normally drive us are mostly negative: financial insecurity if we lived through the Depression; high need for achievement and tangible reflections of that achievement—good cars, homes, kids in college—a conviction that our children no longer consider us wise. Most of us are not, normally, risk-takers.

"You don't have to be what you were before," he says. "You don't have to work in the same industry, do the same job. There are options that seem to be unthinkable when you're caught in the same track year after year." For his clients, it is the pain of termination that creates the need to take a risk. "But voluntarily or involuntarily," he goes on, "it may be time for a good change and your perceptions of that change may well move you into more rewarding work, even at this time in your life."

Time for a change. I thought I was very much alone, one of a kind, when I left the film company in which I was a partner, well over a year ago. The responses from my friends ranged from the comment about having "guts" to "I sure wish I could do it. I envy you." Few were even the least bit pessimistic; most were enthusiastically supportive and optimistic. The remarkable discovery over this past year, though, is the fact that I might consider myself more unusual if I had stayed in the job for ten more years rather than making the move at the age of 57! Far from being alone, I find that I am surrounded by a peer group that is constantly changing, most often for a second career that is not at all connected with the first one.

In *Passages* Gail Sheehy reports the results of a study made by Prof. Judith Bardwick of the University of Michigan, in which every one of the 20 subjects—all outstandingly successful men—had made radical career switches or had become social activists *in middle life!* Why is it that we so often think we are the unusual, the exceptions, only to find, to our surprise, that we are actually one of many?

In a lovely article in *Prime Time* magazine (June 1981), Samuel Schreiner, Jr., wrote of his class of '42 at Princeton. He did not attend the reunion, feeling that he had neither the time nor the money, but in any case he was different in that he had recently resigned from a 20-year job as an editor to pursue a career in writing novels. His assumption was that his classmates would all be at the peak of corporate careers, well settled, well heeled, privileged, and content.

Much to his surprise, a book arrived in the mail and the details of the careers were outlined. He wrote, "I was in for a rude and wonderful shock. Far from being unique, I found that more than 10 percent of my class had opted for new professions, new risks, new lives—in the years when you're supposed to stay put and accumulate juicy pension rights. Not only that, but the entries of all these 'dropouts,' including my own, reflected the joy of rebirth." He also reported that in every case the switch in careers involved reduced income and/or high risk, with a remarkable increase in emotional rewards.

And so it has been for me. For over 35 years I had worked in television and film, the final 15 with three partners in a company that was quite successful in the documentary field. I had garnered my share of awards; my place in the industry was secure. I suppose I had enough of a reputation to continue working in exactly the same way, structuring my life year after year in the same patterns, producing 12 or 15 films each year, accepting the "perks": first-class travel; freedom as an executive; guest lectures at America's universities; and a Fifth Avenue office hung with plaques, testimonials, and my Academy Award nomination. But, something still bothered me.

When I first began the business of making films, I worked with young, vital, and visionary filmmakers, people who would not accept the first solution to a problem. The work was exciting and I was able to spend the time on each project that guaranteed that it would have my very best efforts. Something had changed over all those years and I had become a businessman first and a filmmaker last. Solutions to film problems were too easy; *too much* experience dictated my answers, my thinking, and the eventual product. What had become of the probing, the slow solution to a film problem, working with the young creators who stand at the edges of the motion picture industry, eager to enter?

I suppose I still could have stayed. No one would have known the difference. But my life had taken another turn and my writing of books had begun to be successful. Unlike my college days, when I had filled a scrapbook with rejection slips, my weekend work at writing had begun to show results. After four years there were four books in print and I was living a dual life. I suppose that I should have thought about it for months, mulling over so important a decision in order to give it time to fall into place, but I did not. It took but 24 hours to make up my mind. I called my partners together one Monday morning and I resigned. In one moment I was no longer an executive of the company with which I had worked for so many years. I had cut off the income, the staff relationships, the perks, and a partnership that had worked fairly well, considering that the personalities were so very different.

In a single instant I became an independent filmmaker who wanted to do only two or three films a year for clients whom I liked and respected—and I wanted to do those films as well as I had when I was a young director-producer at the age of 27. I was also, in that single moment, a writer of books in a world that is not known for treating most authors very well financially. In 24 hours I had cleared my office of the memorabilia, the files, the stacked papers, and the funny plaques that hung on the walls ("God So Loved the World, That He Did Not Send a Committee"), 15 years of accumulated junk, birthday gifts from the staff, unnecessary memos, vague corporate letters, and my ash tray that said, "Thank You for Not Smoking." It took nine cardboard cartons to pack what I wanted to keep and take back to my house that could ill-afford to store it all. It took eight more cartons to haul away the old magazines, out-of-date files, and an accumulation of trivia that I had not looked at in 15 years. The day I left, a letter arrived from my dear friend and cameraman Peter Henning, with whom I had worked for 20 years. It read, in part, "Welcome back to the trenches!"

It has been a remarkable year. I was convinced that I would starve and I have not. (The Depression syndrome again.) My old clients have remained with me and I am booked for filmmaking through the middle of next year. There is time to think, time to write, time to escape and fish without feeling the guilt that I have left three partners to fend for themselves. I have been, in fact, busier than ever and the financial rewards have been greater than I had ever expected. And, of course, there has been the readjustment.

I work at home or in my little room on Fire Island and I have had to adjust to being around 24 hours a day rather than going out to an office at 7 A.M. For my wife it has been more difficult, for I am now in "her space" and "her time." The work schedule is of my own choosing and my disciplines are self-imposed, else I would not get anything done. The filmmaking has become a joy again, now that I have put the businessman's hat in the closet and returned to the job of producing films of which I can be proud and in which I have played a vital role. My wife has become active in our small corporation, both in the films and in the books which she has always written, and, since we generally get along well together, my being constantly at home has not been so great a burden as expected—at least not for me.

Our first independent film is due out this week and we are all very proud of it. We have our first full-time employee, Tina Gonzalez, who worked with me at my former company. This small group crowds into an already overcrowded space in a working relationship that is personal, joyful, and productive.

Am I content with the change? The words of Sam Schreiner's Princeton class might well be my own: "Excited beyond my wildest dreams." "I've never regretted the change." A few weeks ago, I walked uptown to an appointment and I began to think. Dodging the New York traffic, I made a list on a scrap of paper, then stopped to sit in a large plaza, using still more paper to compile *three* lists: *The Things I Miss, The Things I Don't Miss, What Has Replaced the Things I Thought I'd Miss.*

I was surprised at the shallowness of the things I missed. Was I really unable to list more than I had, after 35 years? I miss the vitality of uptown Manhattan, though it is there for me to savor, just 20 minutes away, whenever I want to leave my home. I miss the uptown characters, like the man who beats his snare drum on the street. I miss the constant parade of New York women—attractive, well dressed, vital, and so very individual. I miss the perks sometimes, though that feeling is leaving quickly.

I do miss some of the people occasionally, but I have found that corporate divorce is very much like the marital type. It is better for both sides not to keep the contacts alive. And with corporate divorce there are no children, so visitation privileges are not a factor! I do miss the availability of a staff, a full array of people who are there to do my bidding, but I am learning to cope by myself with the aid of my wife and Tina. If I were called upon to detail the one thing that I miss most, I would name the shallowest one of them all. I miss using the company Xerox machine that was right outside my office door! I now have to walk four blocks to take my manuscripts to a small, crowded copy shop. Now *there* is an epitaph for a career of 35 years: *He Misses the Xerox Machine.*

And the things I do not miss? I don't miss the office politics, for you can put any two people together in an office, give them a water cooler around which to congregate, and the lives and loves of all are open to scrutiny and discussion. I don't miss the constant business lunches with people I don't like or with whom I have nothing in common (including the crab grass on their lawns), the aimlessness of conversations at our table or overheard—and no business being done at all, though the main purpose of the luncheon was to discuss "the deal."

I don't miss the routine of the office, though the disciplines are now more severe since they are *my* responsibility. I don't miss being responsible to three other partners and a staff of 22. Though I am running my own business now, and am busier than ever, I don't miss the "businessman" I left uptown at the office.

The things that have replaced it all are diverse, complicated, and new to me. Most of all, the freedom I feel now cannot be equated with anything in my past business life. The decisions, the responsibilities, the rewards are all mine, to be shared only with the people who are immediately around me. My new films show, I think, the effort and the thought that can now go into them. I like to think that I will have more time to expand, to think, to stretch my imagination, but I have been too busy to accomplish any of it yet. My clients are of my own choosing now, and they are people with whom I love to share coffee or a glass of wine in front of the fire or on a terrace that overlooks the entire city. They are people with whom I spend time because I *want* to, rather than because of a sense of corporate duty. After 35 years it is a personal perk that I think I well deserve. And as for the Xerox machine, even that has been replaced with an unexpected dividend. Though the shop is four blocks away, and it is crowded and inefficient, it has become a personal journey each time I take a chapter there for copying. I am now friends with the young man who runs the place, and he comments on each chapter of the manuscript as it goes through the machine. As a matter of fact, it is not even a *Xerox*—I note that he uses a *Kodak* copier! Somehow my copies look even brighter than they ever did before, back at the office!

Soon after the decision to change my life style, the calls and the letters began to arrive from friends, from acquaintances, from clients, from people who had disappeared from my life as much as 10 or 15 years before. One call was from a senior executive of one of America's top ten corporations, a friend whose career I had followed with interest over 25 years as he rose from advertising agency vice-president to a leader in his industry, one quoted in trade journals and lauded for campaigns that feature tunes you and I hum after watching his commercials. Over lunch he informed me that he, too, wanted to change and that my decision had spurred his own. He was retiring at the age of 55 to pursue a second career as a scuba diving instructor! His plan was to take four executives each week to his second home in the Bahamas (flying his own plane to get them there), put them up in his house, and give scuba lessons in the clear blue waters. He would then fly back to pick up another group the following week!

My friend Malcolm went in still another direction at the age of 51. From writing the music for television commercials, a field in which he had developed a superb and rewarding career, he suddenly switched into the nether world of insecurity: Broadway musicals. For him, the catalyst was similar to the reasons so many of us are changing careers at this stage in our lives. "It was not just guts; it was a necessity," he says. "I couldn't look at myself in the mirror. Every time I booked a vacation, maybe once a year, I'd try to gauge when I could safely get away. It's getting to be August. Maybe they'll all be away. Maybe I'll book seven days someplace. So I'd book, take a limo to the airport, but every time, 20 minutes before the flight, after I'd gotten my seat assignment, I'd find a phone and say, 'Did anybody call? Maybe Pepsi, maybe Burger King?' And in the back of my mind I'd have a battle plan. If someone called, I knew where my luggage was, how I could get back into the city. No more. No more. I don't have that any more."

And how has it all worked out? Well, first of all, he has already done the vocal arrangements for a show that is a big hit on Broadway. "The amazing thing is—it's such freedom! When you've spent years doing everybody else's laundry and all of a sudden you've got your own basket and your own clothes, it's a whole different ball game."

A chemical engineer studies law and becomes a public defender, while a middle-aged lawyer becomes a filmmaker. A bank executive leaves the world of finance to strike out as a free-lance writer and in three years has made an indelible mark in the travel field with his books and articles. A public relations director of a large hospital in Memphis opens a small shop that deals in gold and jewelry and in one year moves to the center of the city to expand. A biochemist, who left the field to become a mother and raise two children, returns to school after their teen-age years and becomes the director of a counseling service in California. Possibly the most unusual career change I've heard of recently is that of a successful executive who quit his job at age 50 and went to India to produce pornographic films! You can be certain that his family has used the term "midlife crisis" more than once in describing his move.

And so I am not alone. Many of us are paying no heed to the thinking that we are stalled at middle age, irrevocably mired in the quicksand of routine, security, and the inability to take chances. As longevity increases, more and more of us are looking for a second career, and finding it. Age is no longer a barrier.

A man named James H. Petrie applied to the Moody College branch of Texas A. & M. University in Galveston to train as a merchant marine officer. He was accepted, received a letter of congratulations, and showed up on the campus with a $2,400 federal education loan with which to pursue his career. When he arrived, he was told that the program could not accept him, since the potential of a shipping company employing him was practically nil because of his age. Petrie is 71 years old, plans to sue on the basis of "age-discrimination," and is determined to follow his second career. "I worked on a ship as a teen-ager," he said in an interview. "but I took a different route and I want to find out what I missed!"

One of the most important changes in this century has been the growing numbers of women who are reentering the work force, many of them after the age of 40. Certainly, problems are encountered that are individual and very specific, and I comment on that more fully in Chapter 20. It has been a continuing struggle to achieve equality in a business world run by men. In fact, women earn less money today, as compared to their male counterparts, than they did 25 years ago! In 1955 the earned income of women was about 64 percent of that for men in equal jobs, whereas today it is only 59 percent. The unemployment rates of professionally trained women are two to five times higher than for men in the same field with the same degree of training.

Nevertheless, a dramatic growth in the numbers of women returning to the job market has continued since World War II. The reasons are varied: the sharply declining birth rate; the opening of more jobs for older workers; increased employment opportunities as professions as diverse as firefighter and bank executive are opened (however slowly) to women; divorce and widowhood; and the need for some families to have two breadwinners in order to keep up with the inflation rate, pay the mortgage, the hospital insurance, and the cost of college. Overall there has been a constantly changing attitude toward sexual roles in our society and in the corporate world.

Among the retired, many have found a report by the American

Medical Association to be very true: "There is a direct relationship between enforced idleness and poor health" and the retired are returning to the work force, either in businesses of their own or in volunteer work in the community. Many of our elderly have mixed feelings, however, about being asked to volunteer their services, and I blame them not at all. We all want the dignity of being paid for our work, just as we did when we were younger and beginning the career climb. Nevertheless, if local communities could learn to take advantage of the retired people who want to help, they could increase their total volunteer programs by as much as 50 percent.

In Orlando, Florida, for example, a group of retired persons examined the way in which dependent children were being treated by the juvenile justice system and intervened on their behalf. National organizations such as ACTION (806 Connecticut Avenue, N.W., Washington, DC 20525) and SCORE—Service Corps of Retired Executives—(1441 L Street, N.W., Washington, DC 20416) can give you more information about the volunteer programs in your area.

A short time ago a symposium was held on the subject of "The Future of Older Workers in America," funded by the Work in America Institute, Inc., and the Andrus Gerontology Center of Los Angeles. At a general workshop Jerome M. Rosow, president of the Work in America Institute, made the prediction that "society in the next century will be begging for older workers—there won't be anyone but older workers. They may have to pay them a premium to keep them from retiring." Because of the decline of the birth rate, he feels that by the turn of the century, we will have a work force of which 60 percent will be older workers.

If you add to that the fact that we resent being shunted aside and told that work is no longer important for us—though we have a minimum of 25 productive years still ahead as we reach age 50—there is bound to be a startling change in both the opportunities and the demographics. The stories that we constantly hear and read show that it is already happening. And why not?

We are the elders of the tribe now; we are more experienced, somewhat wiser, and the logical group to be dealing with the problems of our society as well as its productivity. We have been trained in law, corporate structures, medicine, and a thousand other crafts, skills, and professions, not to mention the upbringing of our children and our vast experience in family life. We are men and women who should logically be utilized in jobs that deal with discrimination, functional illiteracy, delinquency, alcohol, and drugs, as well as continuing or changing our careers in the business world if we so choose.

A few evenings ago I sat in the living room of a close friend who has worked for the same corporation for the past 40 years, and who can retire any time he chooses. "I could walk out the company door tomorrow," he says. He would like to be an architect, something for which he was trained as a young man before he was sidetracked, like so many of us, into the corporate world of pragmatism and security. We talked. He looked at me as someone who had done it, who had walked out on 24 hours' notice and was happy about it all. He is wavering, about to make the change. An architect at the age of 62. Why not? Why, indeed, can he not do it? I wait to see what he will do, whether he will gather up that childhood dream and make it work 40 years later. When I left, I told him one of my favorite anecdotes about the change of career in midlife.

Mayor Koch of New York was asked about his chances for reelection and he answered, "If I don't get reelected, the city won't have a better mayor, but I know that I'll get a better job!"

I somehow have the feeling that my dear old friend is going to make an excellent architect!

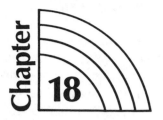

# The Graying of
# the Campus Green

> *I grow old, ever learning many things.*
>
> Solon:
> Fragment 22

It is difficult to believe that the volatile generation of the '60s is more than a decade past. I have always loved to teach, to lecture to young students, to conduct seminars on filmmaking, and to exchange ideas and opinions with the future leaders of my profession. I remember my lectures during that time with a very special sense of joy and excitement, for with all the talk of hippies and flower children and revolution, the students of that period had a dynamism and a probing sense of disbelief that made an establishment professor fair game for their questions, their curiosity, even their rudeness. It was wise to be well prepared for any lecture.

I remember one session at New York University with an undergraduate class in film production. When I entered the room, everyone was reading a newspaper, magazine, or paperback, challenging me to make them put the reading materials away, to give them something important enough to make them listen to *me*. At first I was angry at the lack of respect, for when we went to college, the entrance of the instructor was the signal for immediate attention. Then I laughed and *turned out the lights!* Unable to read any longer, they put the newspapers and magazines aside while a film was shown, and the class was underway.

Question periods were equally exciting and challenging. In a two-hour session, 40 minutes would hardly be enough time to field the queries that ranged from what kind of film stock was used in the documentary to "How can you sell your soul to make films for America's money-grubbing corporations?"

As all things change, this too has changed. The students of the late '70s and the '80s now just sit there and listen. Once again the professor has become God and whatever is given as gospel is written down as such. Well-washed faces look up in blank and accepting trust, and I sometimes feel that if I were to state that "sex is the cause of acne," they would dutifully write it all down in case it came up in the final examination. It is now a waste of time to schedule a long question-and-answer period, for it is generally filled with awkward silences. I began to think that it was *I* who had changed for the worse, until I compared notes with others who teach. The establishment has settled on the heads of our new student generation and it is the *teachers* who are the revolutionaries.

However, there is one area of brightness in all this. During these past four or five years I have been invited to speak to classes and seminars in the field of continuing education, to adults who are holding other jobs while attending school or who have decided to go back to college for a variety of reasons. Some return to improve their chances for advancement in their own professions; some to change careers; some because there has been a smoldering interest in their lives since they were teen-agers, an interest never fulfilled for diverse and personal reasons.

And suddenly, in these continuing education classes all over the country, the age group has changed, and I see before me the faces of men and women who are more mature, more interested, and more concerned with learning as much as they possibly can. It is because they have *chosen* to go to school; for them schooling is not just another unavoidable step in the process of growing up and leaving home. The ages range from about 30 up to the late 70s and even into the 80s. At a recent seminar for adults, the most exciting questions were asked of me by a man of 72 who had always wanted to know more about film directing. This was *his* chance to go back to college! Suddenly, I began to see the vitality of the 1960s without the hostility, in addition to an intensity of motivation and an intellectual stimulation for teacher and student alike.

How rapidly the world of education is changing! And we, as always, are a part of the sudden change. There was a time that we went to school at the age of five or six, graduated from high school or college, then pursued a career until retirement, single-minded, rigidly pro-grammed through our lives, to rust away until death. We were again the victims of a self-perpetuating myth that said that our intelligence and our capacity to learn were declining after the age of 30 or 40. "You can't teach an old dog new tricks," my grandmother used to say. But then she also used to say, "There's no fool like an old fool," and other adages of ageist folklore, too many of them still in circulation today.

How surprised she might be to discover, as the researchers have, that, much to their surprise, there is actual proof of an *improvement* in intelligence and the functions of learning as we age! The *speed* of our performance may decline, but the *capacity* to learn does not di-minish when we have passed the invisible barrier of age 40.

Marty Knowlton, one of the founders of Elderhostel, becomes angry when the subject of waning intelligence is mentioned. In one of our telephone conversations he mentioned the findings at colleges at which Elderhostel classes are conducted. "All of us carry with us that ugly myth that you lose your capacity to learn, that you begin to learn less and less, when in fact the opposite is true. As you get older, you learn better. Experience doesn't diminish the mind; it *increases* your mind. Experience *creates* the mind. Shouldn't your mind be better at 60 than it was at 30?"

Somehow there has been a new liberation in the spirit of learning, of achieving our potential, no matter how late in life, and the return to school by people of our generation has been nothing short of astounding. *More than half* the full-time and part-time college students in the coun-try are adults, and though the term "adult" also includes students from 25 through 45, vast numbers of middle-aged men and women are also returning to the classrooms.

Dr. James C. Hall, dean of University College at Pace University in New York, adds, "Continuing education is just a dynamic view of life. People continue to change. Development doesn't stop at adolescence, and *learning* is a part of development. Continuing education is a function of people developing . . . and not necessarily just in the schools."

Millions of us have gone back to class at community colleges; in our churches and synagogues; in our professional organizations; in our libraries and museums; via television instruction; through correspondence courses; through private lessons in language, the arts, or even tennis; as well as in schools in the armed forces and in prisons!

Colleges and universities began to realize that their enrollments were decreasing as fewer and fewer young people reached the age of entrance. In addition, the dropout rate began to increase. With the alternative of total extinction staring many of them in the face, they began to turn to the adults living right around the perimeters of their campuses, providing new learning experiences for those who wanted to return to school as well as a cushion for the school in the shaky financial times ahead.

Other schools began to realize that changes would have to be made if they were to appeal to the adult student. Our life styles are different from those of college-age students, needless to say. Curricula that took into account the fact that most of us worked during the day, and could not attend classes at normal hours, had to be developed. Administrators had to realize that the usual battery of entrance exams and testing procedures were quite valueless for people who had interrupted their schooling as much as 20 or 30 years before, when college kids like us wore bobby sox. Suddenly there are "weekend" colleges springing up all over the country; morning and evening classes held especially for adult students who commute to work, and new methods of independent study, such as closed-circuit, talk-back television, field work, correspondence study, videotape cassettes, and private tutorial teaching.

Many institutions have removed time limits for completion of degree studies; seminars are being offered at off-campus locations, and at-home study guides now include both writing assignments and examinations. This last is a far cry from our days at college over 30 years ago, when we might sit for three hours, heads bent over minutely printed questions, the proctor or professor stalking the aisles to see that the answers had not been written on our shirt cuffs.

One of the most important innovations that I find, is that most schools and colleges are beginning to acknowledge that our *life experience* is worth analyzing as a prerequisite to reentry into the academic world. Thus we find that many universities are admitting students not only without regard to age, but with a good hard look at such criteria as motivation, creativity, and job history, rather than on the standard college admission guidelines of tests and high school grades.

In his innovative book on nontraditional degrees (*The External Degree*. Jossey-Basse, San Francisco, 1973), Cyril Houle mentions that evaluators are now giving credits for business experience in blueprint reading, writing, management, labor relations, marketing, and cost control, as well as for self-taught skills such as painting and sculpture.

A person who has had 20 or 30 years as a businessman and who is experienced in running a successful company of his own may not have to take preliminary courses, such as Introduction to Business. But Houle also suggests that a man who had farmed for a year might not be qualified in the areas of soil chemistry, and a resident of a city slum would not necessarily have equivalency qualifications for a course in urban sociology.

To be sure, the faculty and the boards of directors of the universities and colleges across the country have not been unanimously enthusiastic about changing the traditional educational processes in order to accommodate the influx of adult students. In spite of the fact that this group has, in many cases, been a financial godsend, the legions of the ivory towers at first resisted the changes, albeit sometimes with good reason. The moment the exploiters of our society began to smell a new market, the diploma mills expanded and the charlatans began their offers of "Surgery Learned at Home" along with other simple programs of instruction! For the legitimate colleges and universities, however, the changes have been a breath of fresh spring air. In all these educational institutions, originally designed for the children and the youth of our society, it is *we* who are preserving the jobs of thousands of professors who had been trapped in a diminishing job market—many of them in our own age group—by this sudden influx of a vital and totally new breed of student. And for those of us of middle age who are the new scholars, the innovations in the educational system have opened up new and exciting horizons. After all these years, we are going back to school!

Henry Seymour, a Pace University student, tells me, "I'm learning as quickly as I did when I got my master's degree in 1937, but it just takes me a little bit longer to write it down when I take an examination." I ask him if it is because he learns more slowly, and he answers with, "No. I just think I'm more *thorough* than I was back in 1937."

He is one of so many. Retired for a year, he is a man who spent 41 years as an international executive with a major pharmaceutical corporation, working and living in Colombia, Ecuador, Venezuela, Mexico, Brazil, and Greece. "There are various reasons that I went back to school. First of all, I don't want to sit and do nothing. Second, I think that the acquisition of knowledge is an end in itself. And third, I want to look around and get a job." His majors are International Business Management and Taxation and he says it is the younger students who turn to *him* for help because the subject is so complicated.

For younger adults, the desire to make more money or to improve their professional positions is what sends most back to school after so many years away from the classroom. Dr. Hall says, "No matter what they tell you, if you probe deeply enough, you find that it's the major reason. However, there are people who have reached a stage in life where they are finally able to pursue something that has always been a second interest in life: physics, astronomy, finance."

Actually only a small percentage of us are going back to school for academic credits or to get a degree eventually, but when we do return for completion of a bachelor's or master's degree we often show ourselves to be superior in both performance and the ability to learn, regardless of age.

The return to school by people of our generation and older also serves to break down the barriers of age-segregation, since the mix of all ages is of benefit to everyone, young or old. The young can learn from the experience of the mature, experienced adult, while the returning student remains in touch with a society that is always in a state of flux, however incomprehensible it may sometimes be to those of us who grew up in simpler and more naive times.

The local high school in Harbor Springs, Michigan, has opened its doors to the elders of the town, and older persons can sign up for any high school class, either for credit or just for fun. Some of the adults are invited to give guest lectures; they share the library, lunchrooms, school band, the classes in microcomputers and ceramics, and most of all the wisdom of years. "Suppose a student is writing a term paper on the lumbering industry in Michigan," a counselor said in an interview. "Imagine how much more alive the material will become to a student when he can sit down and talk to a man who has run a sawmill for 40 years!"

On the college level, possibly the best-known and the ultimate example of intergenerational learning is the Bridge Project of Fairhaven College on the campus of Western Washington State College in Bellingham, Washington. Back in the early 1970s, Fairhaven, like other schools, began to feel the drop in student enrollment. The dean, Ken Freeman, also felt that it was about time to deemphasize the idea that youth is the only time in which to achieve an education. All these years, that attitude was denying the same stimulation for adults of middle age and older.

The original conception called for three groups on the Fairhaven campus in addition to the regular student body aged 18 to 22. The first covered the ages of 2 to 5 in a cooperative day care program for children of students, faculty, and staff, in itself an innovative college plan. The second program provided a support system, including on-campus housing, for reentry students in their later 20s through early 50s who wanted either to prepare for a second career or to move up in the profession they had been pursuing for a number of years. The third group were the adults over 60.

The older students are known around the campus as the "Bridgers," a name given them because their dormitory building is connected to the rest of the school by a walkway, and they are very much in evidence around the lovely campus of Fairhaven. Age-irrelevance is a vital, working idea at the school, and the current director of the Bridge Project, Dr. Douglas Rich, describes the philosophy well. "The fact remains that when we isolate any group of people from the established norm, we usually are contributing to their ill health; however different any group may be, our society is most healthy when such groups remain among us." He quotes Maggie Kuhn's pungent description of age-segregated communities like Sun City as "play pens" that serve only to encourage isolation, robbing people of their social and personal identities.

Participating not only in the formal academic courses like mathematics and philosophy, the Bridgers have thrown themselves into all the extracurricular activities on campus as well—plus the more exotic forms of learning, like belly-dancing and mountain climbing. Of course, there has been readjustment on both sides. One of the elders summed up, "We had stereotyped ideas about 'hippies' and some of our first classes were a shock. I walked into my first math class late. The students were lying all over the floor on their stomachs, on their backs, every which way. I learned soon afterward that the fellow who was sitting in a chair leading the class wasn't the teacher. The teacher was down on the floor with the students! This was a whole new world to me." And another adds, "I'm impressed by how well read the young people are.

When we were in college, all we thought about was whether our shoes and sweaters were in style."

For the younger students it was a revelation to find that the Bridgers were vital and far from over the hill. It has had the additional result of making them unafraid of growing older, and even envious of the attitudes of the elderly students. One of them said, "How very free they are!"

In the area of learning the experience with the Bridge project has been very much like that of the Harbor Springs High School and every other institution that has followed the path of age-integration in its curriculum. The Bridgers make the past seem real. "You can't believe," one youngster comments, "how much more interesting a class in history is when there's an older person in it who has lived through the Depression or who has heard a father or grandfather talk about the time right after the Civil War or World War I."

The experiments in education are continuing all over the country, both in the area of reentry for middle-aged students taking the normal curriculum and in programs specifically designed to bring the older American back into the mainstream of learning—for a degree, for expansion of one's intellectual potential, because of a long-deferred desire to learn, or just for fun. Community colleges in Miami, Los Angeles, and New York, as well as Duke University, Fordham, the University of Maryland, Aquinas College in Michigan, New York University, and Baruch College are just a few of the institutions that have joined the list of innovators.

For those interested in part-time degree programs, there is a publication that gives the information for every area. Published by the National University Extension Association in Washington, D.C., the booklet is called *Who Offers Part-Time Degree Programs* and it's available from Peterson Guides, Book Order Dept., Box 978, Edison, NJ 08817; send $6.00.

The nondegree student who wants to return to school for whatever reason has a choice so vast that no single writer can begin to sort it all out. My office floor is piled high with university and college bulletins that offer courses from The Culture of Morocco, Wraparound and Second Mortgages, Investment Banking, Techniques of Book Editing, and Advertising Workshops to such esoteric and diverse subjects as Psi Phenomena, the Holographic Aspects of Consciousness, I Ching, Tarot Reading, Neighborhood Restaurant Tours, and Beginning Backpacking. All this in addition to "readin', writin', and 'rithmetic"!

Innovations in learning have superceded the boundaries of formal college education. One of the most exciting of these is the group known as Elderhostel, founded in the early '70s by Marty Knowlton and some of his associates. It is based upon the best European tradition of education and innkeeping, but is designed for the elder citizen over 60 who remains active, on the move, and hungry for new knowledge and new friends.

The program is now in all 50 states and Canada and about 20,000 Elderhostelers participate in programs at over 300 colleges and universities. During late spring, summer, and early autumn, when colleges are emptiest and lying dormant, regular members of the college faculty teach a wide range of courses in the liberal arts and the sciences—for example, Practical Alternatives of Solar Energy, Albert Einstein: The Man and the Myth, Philosophy of Religion, Vitality and Fitness, and even a walking tour on The History of Nacogdoches. The catalog listings are marvelous to read. On each campus the Elderhostelers live right in the dormitories, eat in the college cafeteria, and share their schoolwork with other summer students.

It has grown so rapidly that Michael Zoob, vice-president of the nonprofit organization, calls it "the Elderhostel phenomenon" and he says, "It's gone above and beyond the program. It's almost a movement. The hostelers come into the classes with the mental energy and drive professors never see in their undergraduate classes. There are no grades. They don't need the course for a major. They come for no other reason than the love of learning. That's what liberal arts is all about!"

One of the most delightful letters ever received by the group reads as follows:

> *I stumbled on the material about your program in the* New York Times.
> *It met a definite need in me.*
> *I am retired.*
> *I am bored.*
> *I don't know how to play.*
> *I can't settle for gymnastics, crafts, and pep talks* *by 20-year-olds on how great it is to be a senior citizen.*
> *I would still like to be a being in the flow of life.* *Your literature seems to hold out that hope. Do please* *send it to me.*

And the reader of this book might well do the same. Write to: Elder-hostel, Inc., 55 Chapel Street, Newton, MA 02160.

There is a growing hunger to keep learning. When Gay Gaer Luce started SAGE (Senior Actualization and Growth Explorations) in San Francisco, she told me, "We started at 65 and some people started faking their ages in order to get in. So we went down to 60, and then people in their 40s and their 50s wanted to come in. And now there are people who want the training who are in their 20s and 30s. We never intended to isolate older people. What we really wanted to do was to demonstrate beyond a shadow of a doubt that if you did things with the right attitude, it would work whether you were 30 or 90!"

SAGE has been in the forefront of developing a positive attitude toward aging for people who want to explore how growing older can be a rich and creative experience. Quite different from everything else discussed in this chapter, SAGE trains in the areas of relaxation, art and music, gentle breathing and movement exercises through *t'ai chi,* yoga, and meditation.

It represents still another view of aging, a healthy and practical look at ourselves in middle and older age. Dr. Luce explains, "I would have to agree with Jung that the last part of our life has its special purpose. People are not mating. Our culture is immature and for many people the images that the media are broadcasting are the images of the '20s. And so it seems to keep us adolescent forever, always looking for the proper mate. I think there's a real purpose in old age. I think there's a reason that we live long. Its purpose is unfoldment, a spiritual unfoldment, and this is at the core of the radiant health you see in wonderfully developed older people."

Through its educational and outreach programs, SAGE has reached over half a million people throughout the country. If you'd like further information, write to: SAGE, 491 65th Street, Oakland, CA 94609. Dr. Luce's book, *Your Second Life* (Delacorte Press/Seymour Lawrence, New York, 1979) explains SAGE more fully.

For some reason my mini-adventures seem to take place on New York City buses, as described at the very beginning of this book. About four days ago, on the Fifth Avenue bus, a lovely woman in her early 60s sat down next to me and took out what seemed to be a school program. Ever curious, I looked over her shoulder to read, "Institute for Retired Professionals," and I engaged her in conversation to find out where she was heading. The program was begun at the New School in New York in 1962 and membership is open to people who have recently retired from professional or executive careers. It has since spread its innovative thinking to such universities as Harvard, Johns Hopkins, Hofstra, and the University of California at San Francisco and San Diego. For all these retirees, the prime thrust seems to be an indelible restatement of the words of Willard Wirtz: "There must be more to life than 20 years of learning, 40 of earning, and the rest, just waiting!"

I looked with her at her program for that week. Her subjects included German Literature, Hebrew Conversation, Watercolors and Acrylics, and *T'ai Chi!* At 12th Street she spryly leaped off the bus, waved once, and headed down the street to school. Thinking of her program, I mused: Why was I having so much trouble with beginning Spanish? Somehow I could no longer use the lame excuse, "Well, I suppose it must be because I'm getting older!"

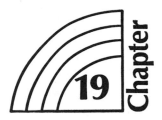

# Madison Avenue
# Discovers Middle Age (at Last!)

> *If there were dreams to sell,*
> *What would you buy?*
>
> *Thomas Beddoes:*<br>Dream Pedlary

**I**f you've spent the greatest part of your working life in the field of selling or marketing or advertising, then I think you will agree with me that we (the author included) have a tendency to develop an ego-centric conceit about the customer. We "know" the buyer from the looker. We can tell the poor from the rich, the bargainer from the impulsive. We are, after all, experienced, with that uncanny perception that comes from the years of dealing with people, and we are—as often as not—*wrong*.

A friend of mine lives in Grand Prairie, Texas, and each year she makes a trip to New York to catch up on the theater, to dine in her favorite restaurants, and to visit some of Manhattan's better stores. She tells of a visit to an exclusive Fifth Avenue department store and the purchase of a new wardrobe for herself and her husband. The young salesman in the shirt department, who also "knew" his customers, had obviously pegged her as an out-of-towner and his hauteur was exceeded   199 only by his obvious indifference and lack of warmth. Her selection completed, she handed him her credit card. He looked up, his suspicions confirmed, and he asked, with a small supercilious grin on his lips, "Grand Prairie? Wherever on earth is Grand Prairie?"

Calmly, she answered, "Oh, it's between Arthur and Irving."

An eyebrow raised slightly, he continued undaunted. "And whatever do you do in Grand Prairie?"

"Oh, we just sit on the porch and watch the oil wells go up and down, up and down!"

Of course, another stereotype took over at once and the word "oil" made the salesman reflect that everyone from Texas is rich and in oil! His manner changed, he whipped out his card and gave it to my friend. "If you ever need help in our store, just look me up!"

It is not at all unusual. Try wearing a pair of faded blue jeans when you visit an exclusive clothing store or you go to buy a custom automobile. Your image will not fit the mold. One of my old dear friends and a longtime client during the 1960s was Rosanne Beringer, president of Welcome Wagon International, over 80 years of age, and one of the most successful executives in the country long before the advent of the token female managers in American industry. She telephoned one day to tell me of an incident that had occurred in the Memphis Lincoln-Mercury showroom, and since the Ford Motor Company was also a client of mine, she thought I'd be interested. I was.

"Young man," she indignantly sputtered. (She always called me "young man" when she was angry.) "Young man, you should call those clients of yours at once and tell them this story!" She had gone into the dealership with her daughter, wanting to purchase a brand new Lincoln. She looked, she touched, she sat in the seat, she handled the wheel, and all the while not a single salesman came over to assist her. For over half an hour, ignored by the staff, she looked at the car. Finally, angry and distressed, she left, walked across the street, and purchased a Cadillac!

To the salesmen she "obviously" was not a buyer. *No woman of 80* walks into a dealership ready to whip out a checkbook and pay cash for a brand new luxury car! In the sagacity of their conceit, the salesmen had pegged her as a "tire kicker"—a looker, but not a buyer. Had the prospect been a well-dressed *man* of 80, he would have been duly pegged as a wealthy, retired chairman of the board of a major corporation, and the rush to serve him would have mauled fifteen salesmen in the stampede!

To those who claim to reflect the images of our society—the advertising community, the marketers, the purveyors of communications—two entire generations (ours) have been dismissed for a long time as "tire kickers." I have discussed our invisibility in the media in Chapter 6. Until now the advertisers have considered us so unimportant in their scheme of "cost per thousand" that we do not even exist in the mailing lists! A group that is now active in the furtherance of the rights of women looked desperately to purchase a list covering ages 45 to 65, and nowhere could one be found! Certainly they could have acquired lists for the aged, adolescents, college students, middle-income liberals or conservatives, gun owners, gun haters, and cat fanciers, but the demographics did not exist for "Women, Age 45–65."

But if the face of aging is changing, so possibly is the awareness of the advertising community. Every so often the sleeping giant of Madison Avenue, comatose in Rip Van Winkle isolation these past 20 years, is shaken awake by discovery and revelation. The *Harvard Business Review* has published an article by Rena Bartos, a senior vice-president at J. Walter Thompson, titled "Over 49: the Invisible Consumer Market." Stephen J. Frankfurt, an old friend from my early television and film days, and now the director of creative planning at Kenyon and Eckhardt, has effectively spoken and written to his industry on "The Maturity Market"—us—the people from age 45 to 64. Suddenly, from a state of sheer invisibility, so long neglected, too often insulted, perpetually ignored, we are beginning to be discovered as "active affluents" or "active retireds." Why? Why have we gone so abruptly from the back door of the marketplace to become the fair-haired, albeit rapidly graying, favorite children of the business community? The reasons, of course, are simple and what surprises me is that it took so long to discover them:

> There are lots and lots of us and we are growing rapidly as a group.
> *We have lots of money!*

We are growing at a faster rate than any other segment of the population, while the youth generation is shrinking. At the time of this writing, our numbers are vast and awesome. We are *44 million* people, aged 45 to 64, almost twice the *total* population of Canada—more people than the combined citizenry of all the Scandinavian countries with Austria and Belgium thrown in! All those millions of people and yet,

until now, the attitude of Madison Avenue has been that our buying
habits were established during our own years in the "Pepsi generation"
and they cannot change now. As Hubert Pryor, editor-in-chief of *Modern
Maturity* magazine, put it, "Clearly, if that were the case, everybody
in the maturity market today would be using Kolynos toothpaste, driving
an Essex, reading *Liberty,* and drinking sarsaparilla."

What is more important, perhaps, is the fact that the attitudes
of the 45–64-year-old age group make us consumers the likes of which
the advertising world has never quite seen before. We have postponed
much of our lives until now—the children had to be diapered, raised,
schooled, and prepared for the world. For the most part they have gone
to lead their own lives. For the first time we do not have to make
sacrifices for them. Steve Frankfurt, in a speech before the Western
States Advertising Agencies Association in Monterey, California, commented on the continuing erosion of "the Puritan, work-oriented ethic"
and stated that we are becoming more self-indulgent, putting more
emphasis on "having it now." He went on to say, "For the first time
since taking on the responsibilities of marriage, the couple is free to
think about themselves, what *they* want or need, how *they* want to
spend their money, what kind of car *they* can now have." He calls it,
rightly, "mom-and-pop time"!

In spite of the myths about us, we are in excellent health for the
most part, and are reported to watch our waistlines and diets more than
any other age group. Less than 1 percent of us are listed by the census
takers as being seriously ill. We are, in fact, the greatest single market
for luxury items and for travel, even if we don't appear too often in the
ads. Last year I produced a film on a cruise from Vancouver to Alaska
and fully 85 percent of the passengers on the ship were in our age
group or older! We also demand more luxury in our travel. We've put
our backpacks away forever.

We actively buy a thousand or more product categories that range
from swimming pools to investments, from boating equipment to restaurant dinners, from second homes to credit cards; magazines and
newspapers, luggage, and automobiles. In fact, the 45–64-year age
group is more apt to own two, and even three, cars than any other
segment of the population.

We represent a market that is worth over $300 *billion*—53 per-
cent of the country's buying power—to manufacturers and advertisers
alike, yet it has taken so long for them to discover us. We have more
discretionary income and spending power than younger or older age
groups; almost 90 percent of us own our own homes, three-quarters of

us have savings accounts; we love to entertain; we're active in gardening, fishing, bicycling, tennis, camping, and photography. And I note with interest a statistic in the *Harvard Business Review* article that we "not only invest in stocks and bonds, [but] are the only segment above the norm for buying diamond rings." *Sarsaparilla and* Liberty *magazine indeed!*

The perpetuation of our invisibility becomes even more appalling if we read still further to find out just who we are and how much potential we do have, not only in the marketplace, but in every facet of our lives, economic as well as political.

> ▰ The per capita income in the 45-to-54-year age group is about 12 percent higher than the national average. When we look at the bracket between 55 and 64, per capita income rises to 26 percent above average.
> ▰ About 30 percent of all households in America are headed by people who are in the 45-to-64-year age group. In terms of numbers, it translates to approximately *25 million people.*
> ▰ With the children gone and more time available for other pursuits, there are more wage earners per household than in the younger segments of the population and, concomitantly, more earners than dependents.

There is, of course, a very real danger in this new discovery of our generations as an affluent, vital, active part of the consuming public. It might well hurt the elderly poor and affect our own entry into the ranks of those over 65 in these next few years. The myth of every aging person subsisting on a diet of dog food is slowly giving way to still another pernicious distortion, and I have begun to read about it in popular magazines like *Newsweek* and in the special interest business publications. This new myth portrays *everyone* over the age of 50 as affluent and totally independent. America has gotten rid of the poor forever!

An article in *Forbes* magazine tried to debunk the idea that a large number of our elderly are in need of help from the government, a growing attitude in these days of "too much government control over our lives." By using selective and exceptional cases (which every author uses, of course), *Forbes* gives the distinct impression that we are *all* well heeled, living in the lap of luxury, buying condominiums and sailboats, and becoming filthy rich in the stock market.

I sense in this shifting perception of an entire group a potentially harmful result, equally as damaging as the myth that we are all in penury. Certainly most older Americans are better off today than they were 10 or 15 years ago, and I have spent much of this chapter detailing the statistics. But as Cyril F. Brickfield, executive director of the American Association of Retired Persons, has written, "Normally, we would welcome the efforts of those who seek to correct misconceptions about older citizens. But the new myth makers go too far. Rather than just explode the old stereotypes, they are creating new ones. They are implying that because the elderly have made substantial gains, they can now afford to make major sacrifices, such as giving up some of the cost-of-living protection provided by Social Security." It is a critical and sobering view for those of us who are now in middle age and who represent the affluence of which I've written.

Like you, I try to balance my feelings of being a part of this affluent generation of ours with my conscience and continual awareness of the social problems with which I grew up. I do enjoy my role in an age group that is overall less dependent upon others than are the very young and the very old. At the same time, I look with admiration, faith, and some dependence upon the people who will be described in the following chapter, to make certain that the myths of middle age and the elderly are destroyed forever, but without being replaced by other societal straitjackets that reflect the self-interests and narrowness of those whom we elect to govern us, those who communicate to us, or those who merely try to sell to us their products.

If we are a newly discovered market, I will revel in it and smile as the "Pepsi generation" on television seems to be turning gray, or as I note the *Wall Street Journal* headline that advises its readers, "Advertisers Start Recognizing Cost of Insulting Elderly." It is not all bad and I shall accept it for now, waiting suspiciously for a change of fickle heart by Madison Avenue should they discover another group to love. For the moment, it will do. My mother loved me as her son, good or bad, my wife "in sickness and in health," my German shepherd dogs for my loyalty and devotion. Thus when *Harvard Business Review* ends its article with, "If we get off the comfortable rocking-chair way we have always defined our targets, we might discover significant opportunities within the invisible consumer market," I am overjoyed with my new experience. I am finally being loved for *my spending power!*

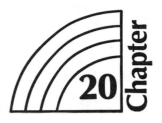

# Man (Person) the Barricades!

> *You're wrinkled babies! Sniveling! You're the eld-*
> *ers of the tribe. What are you doing for the tribe's*
> *survival?*
>
> *Maggie Kuhn*

I remember it as a rainy day in April. I had come into New York from my island especially to attend the meeting, and the warmth of the YWCA lobby in midtown Manhattan felt comfortable in the early spring chill. Convinced in my usual grumbling pessimism that I would be the only person to show up on a day like that, I was pleasantly surprised to see the milling, vital women who had already arrived, shaking off umbrellas, picking up pamphlets, signing the register. A charming registrar came up to me and asked if, perhaps, I might be in the wrong place. No, I told her, checking my folder, I assumed that this was the meeting of the Older Women's League? She nodded, smiled again, and went back to her desk.

The huge hall was packed, rain notwithstanding, with probably over 400 women, attractive, alive with a humming anticipation, all of them between the ages of 45 and 65. Four hundred women—and me. For I realized, looking around, that I was the only man present, an obvious fact brought home still further when the meeting began and Jo Turner of the OWL National Board greeted the group with, "Good afternoon, sisters," then, turning to look directly at me, "and *brother*!"

It has been a long time since that rainy afternoon and I have watched with interest as groups like OWL have sprung up, expanded, increased their political power, and made themselves heard in a world that continually strives to keep our generations invisible. Suddenly, too, I have watched with awe as middle-aged men and women have begun to protest, very loudly, very effectively, not only through their organizations but also as individuals, as busload by busload they have become the massed verbalization of the things that threaten us most.

In September of 1981, a quarter of a million people marched, drove, and bused to Washington, D.C., in a protest that was to become known as Solidarity Day, and the faces were not the same as those we saw in the '60s. Not at all. One man, about 50 years old, wearing a hard hat, sat on the Mall and commented, "I thought the protest marches were for kids who had too much time on their hands. They'd come down here, have riots, smoke marijuana, and tear down the system." There were many middle-aged faces in Washington on that day, for there was a threat in the minds of the protesters that everything they wanted, everything they had worked for, was under fire from an administration that didn't quite understand—or care. And so they marched, these brothers and sisters of middle age. How times have changed!

And I think I have changed too, and that I have grown these past years, for I have become more aware of the multiplicity of problems, the almost insurmountable odds in the struggle for equality regardless of age or sex, the reemergence of new social concerns just as we think we have made headway against the old ones.

I think I have been awed and impressed, too, by the fact that this past year has opened new feelings, new determination, and the surprising discovery that, for the most part, it is the *women* who are leading the battle on ageism, while we men lag far behind in our activism. Possibly, too often, the male has been involved with his career, confident that nothing will ever change, that life will continue as it has, that problems cannot affect us while under the umbrella of a male-dominated, male-oriented legislative and corporate world. And then, one day, the roof falls in and we are shocked and surprised and cast adrift. Is it because the women, on the other hand, have always been discriminated against in the society—economically, socially, and legislatively? Finally their voices are being heard. And it might be well for all of us to listen.

"It's a call to political action," Maggie Kuhn says, "but not as vested interests, not as a self-serving group. It's a call to a new kind of political responsibility for the survival of society . . . because *age* is a universalizing force and a universal human experience. Not all of us are black, not all of us are women, not all of us are minorities. But we're all getting *older*!"

When she was 65, Maggie Kuhn was forced to retire from the editorship of a church magazine. Wounded and angry, she fought back and she gathered five friends to form an organization that would battle to change the laws, as well as the attitudes, that make up a pattern of age discrimination in our country. It was the press that teasingly referred to the tiny group of battlers as the "Gray Panthers" and the name stuck. A decade later, there are about 50,000 members in the Panther network, with about 110 local groups that transcend all ages. As a matter of fact, more than *half* the membership is under 65, ranging from teenagers to a large segment of people in our generation.

I suppose that too many of us think that the "barricades" of our youth, the battles fought for social concerns and what we considered justice, are long gone; that it doesn't do much good to fight the establishment anyway, and that we're "getting too old" to do combat on the field of communal interests. Maggie is now in her late 70s and, when I spoke with her in Philadelphia, I asked to see her schedule for the next month. She makes more than 200 speeches a year and the following week was to appear at the University of Pennsylvania Medical School, before the Congressional committee on Social Security in Washington, then in New York for a meeting of a United Nations committee planning a world assembly on aging. Friday night of that week she was to make still another speech before a group of accountants working in the public interest, and on Saturday she'd be in Minneapolis-St. Paul for yet another appearance.

"Don't you ever get tired?" I asked.

"Yes, I do. I get very tired," and she drew herself up, this diminutive dynamo of a woman, and said, "but I plug into the energy of the groups and I get energized from them!"

If you or I were to comment on Maggie's age, she would probably put us down with the fact that Susan B. Anthony was 84 when she culminated her lifetime battle by organizing the International Women's Suffrage Alliance in Berlin. Margaret Mead remained a dynamic, strong, vocal force well into her 70s. The list is endless.

The important question, of course, is: Does it do any good? The Gray Panthers have been active in *all* the areas of society, not just in the field of aging: antiwar, antinuclear, the basic right of affordable housing, adequate health care, racism, sexism, and all the forces that demean and dehumanize people, regardless of age. Protest *is* an effective weapon.

> 🖉 Under pressure from the Gray Panthers, Congress raised the permissible mandatory retirement age from 65 to 70. They are also promoting new work force concepts—job-sharing, phased retirement, sabbatical leaves, and midcareer changes to allow people to work at any age.
>
> 🖉 A four-year study of nursing homes exposed the shocking conditions that prevail in so many of them; there are Panther networks monitoring their own local nursing homes and the agencies responsible for enforcing reforms. They are also seeking alternatives to placing our elderly parents in institutions, for they believe as I do that 40 percent of nursing home patients could live successfully in their own communities if homemakers, hot meals, and minimal health services were provided.
>
> 🖉 Their class-action suit against the Federal Reserve System has resulted in higher passbook rates for small savers, most of whom are elderly.

The Gray Panthers are also involved, along with other organizations, in fighting the proposed cuts in Social Security, lobbying for comprehensive national health insurance, consumer protection, and intergenerational housing.

The latter theory is practiced by Maggie herself. "Our rigid age-segregation—the 'ghettoization' of young and old people—is contrary to the larger public interest," she says. "Ultimately it will destroy the sense of community when you have more and more old people living in isolation. I think if you've been to Sun City, it's horrible, and it's the same in parts of Florida."

She now lives in a large, sprawling house in Germantown, which she shares with two women in their 30s, a man of 28 and three large cats. Maggie comments, "This living together of young and old is just what our society needs. Today, young people scarcely get to see an old person up close—until they become one themselves!"

Unfortunately, the idea is not an easy one on which to expand. Though it has worked in some areas, including an experiment at Bucknell University (in which older students returning to college shared living quarters with the younger ones), much of the zoning in the

United States prohibits more than two or three unrelated people from sharing living quarters. In Yugoslavia, the *komencias* provide older persons without relatives the support of a younger family of their choice. The agreement provides care to the older person until death, at which time the property and estate are inherited by the younger people. It is a subject that is gaining acceptance here in the United States, especially in times of very tight housing and a runaway inflation rate. We may all see the day in which surrogate families begin to play an important role in the aging process. Maggie says, "I cannot tell you how many times I have quietly thanked God for my good fortune at having Linda, Bob, and Bobbie as my housemates, and dear friends."

Of course, *I* am now a Gray Panther and proud of it! The membership fee is minimal; the newspaper, *Network,* gives me joy and keeps me up to date, and I am still constantly amazed by the fact that Maggie's schedule has not let up one bit! If you'd like information, write to the Gray Panthers at 3635 Chestnut Street, Philadelphia, PA 19104.

There is much in the fight to gain our rights, to be heard in our crying out for equitable treatment, that stirs a faint undertone of ambivalence in me. I have always considered myself a battler when the need arose, though living in a world where evenhandedness and compromise are often needed to survive or to achieve even a small measure of success. I have written my letters to the editors, to corporations, and to my Senators, most often without success, sometimes with notable recognition. However, I have found that too often the lone voice of dissent is easily squelched, while the strength of an organization or a programmed campaign is triumphant through the powerful voice of sheer numbers.

My ambivalence occurs when I roundly condemn the people who think differently of using pressure tactics when they develop a strong following of activists to convince the networks, for example, that certain types of "jiggle" programs and TV violence are unsuitable for the chaste American family. On the other hand, I strongly support the groups and organizations that are pressuring these same networks to end their silent support of ageism, sexism, and racism. I accept my hostility and my anger with "the other side" because I feel that they preach censorship and boycott, though they deny it vehemently. Then I look to myself and ask why I am any different when I refuse to buy the products of a manufacturer because of the company's role in supplemental infant feeding or in the delivery of dangerous birth control devices to third-world countries. Am *I* then not supporting a boycott? Of course I am.

But is it not natural to think that *they* are unfair and that *we* are right, while they think that *we* are unfair and *they* are right? At times like these I merely set my stubborn jaw and mutter the line from Voltaire, "Your freedom ends where my nose begins," and I go back to do battle, firmly convinced that *they* are wrong and *we* are right!

At the meeting of the Manhattan chapter of the Older Women's League, Natalie Priest, a superb actress and chairman of the AFTRA (American Federation of Television and Radio Artists) Women's Committee, asked a question of the audience:

"How many of you saw the Oscar broadcasts the other evening?"

Several hands went up. I was surprised at the small response, since I was convinced that *everyone* else watched Hollywood's inflated image of itself, even if I didn't. She went on.

"Did you notice the absence of anything in the commercials? Do you realize that there was *not one single older woman* in a commercial in a broadcast that was 2½ or 3 hours long?"

Earlier in the book I devoted an entire chapter to the problems of the media and just why I consider them an enemy of the aging. This is a prime area in which strong protests are being mounted by groups interested in halting the stereotypical, distorted images and the omissions of older people, and older women in particular, from network programs and commercials.

The Gray Panthers, always in the forefront, have had a National Media Watch Committee since 1973, administered by a remarkable woman in her late 70s, Lydia Bragger. Culling information and research from viewers all across the country, they have been meeting with network officials and advertising agency executives, the National Association of Broadcasters, and the select committees of the Congress of the United States. They use blowups, film clips, and transcripts of programs and commercials, and they document their complaints with the figures acquired from their watchers across the country. In addition, the Universities of Georgia and Maine have developed courses on media-watch monitoring.

AFTRA and Equity, in conjunction with the Women's Action Alliance, a consortium of women's groups all over the country, formed their project to make women aware of how they were (or were not) being represented on television and radio. More than 40,000 commercials were monitored—38,000 on television and 2,500 on radio in 41 states—by over 450 women in 71 organizations. The results, as I reported earlier in this book, certainly were no surprise to anyone. The older woman is the least represented category in the entire world of commercials. "We are confined," Natalie Priest says angrily, "to doing an occasional ad for hemorrhoids, false teeth, and Geritol!"

Progress has been slow but the protest letters to the networks and the agencies have begun to pay off. Some Colgate-Palmolive commercials now show that older people take showers just like younger ones. People like Mollie Parnis, the designer, and Anne Jackson, the actress, have done on-camera work. The fact is that the networks and the agencies do pay attention to the mail they receive. (Look at some of their horrified reactions to "the other side.") AFTRA has suggested a program of "Orchids and Onions"—letters written to the television station, the manufacturer, or the advertising agency. Send an "orchid letter" when you want to praise them, or an "onion letter" if you've got a gripe. Most local stations are listed right in your telephone directory and all products have mailing addresses on their labels.

Don't expect miracles, but take the time to write anyway. And keep in mind that the advertising agencies and the television industry are the same as the rest of the corporate world; they are run almost entirely by men. Some of them are sensitive to the invisibility of older women; some are totally insensitive. For example, at a recent meeting of the American Association of Advertising Agencies in New York, the audience numbered about 400; all but 40 or possibly 50 were men. Of the 22 speakers who served as the voices of the industry at that meeting *one* was a woman. With odds like those, why should the *men* be angry?

For the male of my generation it is difficult (but I hope, not impossible) to shed the cloak of chauvinism. Brought up in an era when the roles of gender were carefully drawn, it was the *man* who supported the family, as did our fathers and our grandfathers, while the woman remained at home to nurture, to tend, and to mother. We men may give lip service to the idea of equality, but too often it is lacking in our actions, even today. It is very much like Jim Gallagher's story of the Navy petty officer who stormed, "I don't care how many changes they make around here, as long as they don't do things differently than they've been doing them!"

As Dr. Elizabeth Most, a retired professor of social work, said in a speech to OWL members, "Being married generally meant isolation from the world outside and having practically complete responsibility for home and the rearing of children. . . . Magazines gave us an idealized picture of ourselves. . . . They presumed that we could accomplish miracles in the home on no matter what budget and yet present ourselves of an evening relaxed and ready to seduce the husband." There was, of course, laughter at this point. Then she went on: "From childhood on, we perceived ourselves through the eyes of men . . . a perception of inferiority and self-abasement, for along with the rhetoric and the pedestal, the reality was scullery work for most older women!"

Consider that most women spend 20 or more years in the administration of the household, management of the family budget, supervision of the cuisine, directing the "client relations" involved with entertaining business guests who are suddenly there for dinner, serving as purchasing agent for everything from the weekly groceries to furniture, doubling as transportation captain for the kids and the friends of the kids, being the doctor, nurse, and paramedic, as well as executive vice-president of the family. What happens when such a woman comes out into the marketplace *run by men* to look for a second career? She is considered *unskilled*. Unskilled, middle-aged, and relegated to the lowest-paying jobs, while the men are just reaching the height of their careers at the ages of 40 or 50!

I have a sometime fantasy in the form of a short playlet in which the normal love relationship leading to marriage is replaced by a job interview, much as it would be in a corporation. The homemaker applicant sits before the male interviewer, hands demurely clasped on her lap, her legs together, hair combed neatly.

*SHE:* What does the job entail?

*HE:* I'm offering you a position as "homemaker." You'll have to clean, shop, plan, be nice to my mother and father, be the social hostess, give birth to the babies, stay at home and care for them while they're young, be nice to my boss, keep the checkbook balanced . . .

*SHE:* (interrupts) What does the job pay?

*HE:* (baffled) Pay?

*SHE:* I mean, what is the salary, what are the perks?

*HE:* (annoyed with the effrontery) Well, it doesn't pay any *money*. What I'm offering is a lifetime job with security, a chance to be a companion, a helpmate. We don't demean the job with *money!*

*SHE:* (rises and begins to leave) I think I'll look somewhere else!

It doesn't take a feminist to understand, then, why organizations like the Older Women's League are forming. Through a reevaluation in middle age, or through divorce or widowhood or just plain free choice, a woman discovers that she is on very shaky financial ground. An angry woman rises at a meeting and recounts her own experiences: "We've been out of the job market for years. We go to an employment agency and they say, 'Where is your résumé?' *We have no résumé,* except for having successfully, I hope, raised a family!"

The Older Women's League is attacking three major areas of inequity through its more than 25 chapters throughout the country:

*Social Security Benefits.* There are both built-in inequities in the system, such as the husband being eligible for full benefits while a surviving wife must live on a minimal payment, and proposed reductions that will severely affect the older woman.

*Pension Rights.* Again, the male breadwinner is entitled to full benefits—until he dies. The widow is generally left with nothing or with very little, even though she has worked all her life at raising the family so the husband could devote his efforts to the job. All divorced wives of government workers, railroad workers, military men, and foreign service personnel are left stranded. The laws of inheritance in the farming industry have forced surviving wives to sell the farms in order to pay taxes, in spite of the years of working alongside the husband in the fields and in the barns, and while tending the kitchen alone.

*Access to Health Insurance.* This is an area that is usually tied directly to employment and, in many cases, to age. Divorced or widowed, a woman generally cannot acquire the same coverage as that held by her spouse, and conversions are very expensive.

The common thread of all three problems is that there is a cry to recognize the value of women's work, paid or unpaid; to focus on the economic plight of women in their later years, and to attack the inequities in public policy. Jean Phillips, who heads her own public relations firm, is president of the Manhattan chapter of OWL. She formed the group, only 18 members at first, and then, "The response we've had to this definitely indicates that this is an idea whose time has come. There was an article in the *New York Times* and the woman who wrote it told me that she's never had such response to anything she's ever written in her entire life. We've been inundated with letters and calls; we have a mailing list of about a thousand people from all over the country, from Canada, even from Switzerland and South America. They say, all of them, 'oh, this is so great, we feel that we've been neglected . . . that nobody cares . . . that we're over the hill . . . and we just think it's time that we're heard.' "

At OWL there are no age limitations, even though the organization was formed for women between 45 and 65. There is one woman of 87 who is a member, and so are her 57-year-old daughter and her 29-year-old granddaughter. "A lot of young women want to join us," says Jean Phillips. "They say, 'I can see myself in a few years!' They say that it's been bad for their mothers and *they* don't want to end up that way."

The membership fee is very nominal, and you can get further information about the chapter of the Older Women's League in your area by writing to them at 3800 Harrison Street, Oakland, CA 94611.

For women reentering the job market after divorce or widowhood, another source of help and guidance is the Displaced Homemakers Network, Inc., 755 8th Street, N.W., Washington, DC 20001. Their *Program Directory* provides a listing of centers, programs, and projects around the country that offer services to the displaced homemaker. Their newsletters to members are further sources of information on reading materials, new books, films, conferences, and current legislative issues of interest to older women.

For women who want legal advice on marriage and divorce, women's health services, women's centers, as well as counseling advice and information, skilled trades training centers, and women's commissions, the Women's Action Alliance has just published a new and comprehensive directory. It's called *Women Helping Women: A State by State Directory*, and it's available from Neal-Schuman Publishers, Inc., 23 Cornelia Street, New York, NY 10014. At the time of this writing, the cost is $14.95.

We are, none of us, valiantly fighting the battle alone. Not by any means. There are also large and effective organizations with memberships in the hundreds of thousands—and, indeed, in the millions—which are also involved in the struggle against ageism. Possibly they don't have the "personality" of the groups I've mentioned, but they do have the clout of the establishment and the knowledge and experience in Congressional lobbying that most of us lack as individuals. Many have been fighting the conservatism and the rigidity of organizations like the American Medical Association—which was against Medicare when it was first brought to the floor of Congress and which has been against other programs of national health insurance that might aid the elderly and the indigent. Americans for Democratic Action has joined the battle for equal pay for women. Many of the groups listed below have raised their voices on the issue of the integrity of Social Security. And now we are beginning to hear the massed voices of the unions; the National Association for the Advancement of Colored People; the National Organization of Women; Republicans, Democrats, and Independents. We are not, by any means, alone!

The National Retired Teachers Association and the American Association for Retired Persons have a membership of over 13 million, and the National Council of Senior Citizens numbers 3 million. There are others, including the National Association of Retired Federal Employees, the American Association of Homes for the Aging, the National Council on Aging, and the National Caucus on the Black Aged. For the middle-aged reader who does not want to get personally involved in the activities of groups like the Gray Panthers or OWL, or who does not yet want to march on Washington, these larger groups provide an outlet through membership, and no matter how small an effort that seems, it is important in this battle that affects us all.

If we are aware of the societal treatment of the middle-aged and the elders—and how can we not be aware?—if we are not to be relegated to the status of second-class citizens in a culture that reveres and idolizes youth; if we are not to be pushed aside when we reach the age of 45, we *must* speak up, each of us.

We *must* make ourselves heard, else *we* remain the first and foremost enemy of our own age group! There is so much to do. We vote in larger numbers than our younger citizens, who still do not understand the democratic process fully. We have isolated the problem of our invisibility by becoming aware of the myths and angry at the stereotypes, many of which we have been carrying firmly within our own heads. We even have the support and the good will of many of the young people, else they would not join us as we raise our voices along with those of the Gray Panthers and the other so-called "older" groups. Most of all, we are beginning to evolve a sense of self.

Certainly it is frustrating when we are surrounded by so many groups with their own self-interests and their voices that clamor to be heard. The farm lobby and the tobacco lobby and the gun lobby and

the continual filibusters on budget, defense, foreign policy, high interest, and inflation continue to fight for the daily headlines, while we
sometimes feel that our thin voices are being drowned out by a ca-
cophony of political jukeboxes. Of course, it is no fun to fight and lose.
It is sad to put energy and time and thought and emotional strength
into the battle, only to find that we are not being heard even half the
time. It is difficult to start all over again, right from the beginning. But
it is the quality of our survival for which we fight. It would be truly sad
if we refused to fight at all.

# Epilogue
# Chrysalis Awakening

"Unlike the kids who are trying to find out who they are and what the world is all about, we *know*—we've been there. Over the years we've stockpiled knowledge, experience, and good sense, and we're set to put them to good use. In ways no other midlife generation has known before, we are active, involved, and venturesome, with the capacity for enjoyment that few youngsters can ever know. ... *At last it's time for me!*"

Barbara V. Hertz, Publisher
*Prime Time* magazine
(August 1980)

It is, perhaps, more difficult to end this personal accounting of a journey than it was to begin it, when hundreds of empty white pages lay in wait beside my restless typewriter. For, as the days and the weeks 217 have passed, and the anniversary of more than a year of writing went by unnoticed, I realized that this discovery of middle age would continue to unfold unabated, even as the chapters were concluded and long after the book was published.

Is it just that *I* have become more aware, more observant, of the continual growth and vitality of our generations, more cognizant of *us* as a very special group of people? Before this book, and in my own personal way, had I also been infected with the virus of invisibility and self-doubt in a country that venerates youth—until I began to analyze more carefully just what it is that has been infecting our entire society?

Not once in this year have I discovered what might be described as *typical of us;* not once could I determine just when we turn from "young" to "middle-aged" to "elder" with all the myths and all the stereotypes that the labels connote. We are so often concerned with dividing our lives into chronological segments that we violate the concept that living has an essential *wholeness,* a continuum in which the same social, psychological, and economic factors that affect us as young people are still with us all through our adult lives. As the great baseball pitcher, Satchel Paige, so wisely inquired, "How old would you be if you didn't know how old you was?"

In the writings of the Talmud, of Confucius, and of the Greek poet and lawmaker Solon, we read again and again that the years of middle age— from 40 to 65—allow the greatest potential for proficiency and achievement, the greatest contributions to society, the greatest fulfillment in terms of our capabilities and our interests. And though Confucius and Solon set longevity at age 70, the Talmud wisely foresaw our longer life span and recounted our virtues until the age of 100, with a mere 50 as the time for giving counsel and 60 for wisdom. I am reminded of the blessing given by my grandmother and others in my family as they intoned, "You should only live and be well until 120!" Even the 100 years of the Talmud were not enough for her!

The ancient sages were not wrong. If we probe deeply, we find that middle age has not altered our perception of ourselves as individuals. Except for the inevitable physical changes, we are not much different from the way we were in our youth. Often we find that life has turned out much better than societal myths have led us to expect, and we think of ourselves as the *exceptions* rather than the *examples* of millions who feel and think and react and enjoy life in a freedom of spirit that only comes with reaching our middle years!

We look around, and suddenly it is a time when the children are grown and on their own. Suddenly oft-postponed pleasures are there within our grasp. Suddenly it is a time to enjoy the family while maintaining a sense of freedom, the likes of which we have never experienced before. It is, for most of us, finally, a time of stability and financial independence. But most of all, perhaps, it is a time when we begin to understand our own wisdom and our own maturity. Bernice Neugarten calls it "the conscious processing of new information in the light of what one has already learned and the turning of one's own proficiency to the achievement of desired ends." She concludes with the thought that it is a time when we begin to create our own rules and our own norms.

Eleanor Roosevelt, on her 77th birthday, was heard to say, "Life was meant to be lived. Curiosity must be kept alive. One must never, for whatever reason, turn his back on life." Interestingly, in this past year, I have found that very few of us *have* turned our backs. Quite the contrary—the vast majority of us have just begun to discover ourselves in ways that we might never have thought possible.

When I left Maggie Kuhn that rainy day in Philadelphia, the interview over, Maggie fluttering from desk to desk, taking calls, having her next speech copied, we stopped for one last hug of goodbye. The fire was in her eyes again and she spoke of *now*. "Now you can finally say what you want to say and no one will berate you. You can say it in the way you want to say it and no one will scold you. Now . . . it's a time for *now*!" It was not until weeks later that I found a similar uplifting line in *Passages,* in which Gail Sheehy wrote, "The motto at the stage past 50 might well be 'no more bullshit!' "

And, thus, in this past euphoric year of discovery, I have begun to listen to the voices around me, to hear the chorus of people of middle age who have suddenly realized that we have spent far too much time trying to be what society thought we should be, trying to be younger if youth demanded it, trying to be more agreeable if our children nagged about it, trying to fit the mold of everyone else's idea of who we are and how we should feel and what we should think. As Gae Gaer Luce wrote, "We victimized ourselves and blamed our age."

Look around you, as I have done. Listen carefully, for we have much to say that is worth hearing. We are really terribly attractive; we are certainly more interesting than we were at the age of 20! I walk into an elevator in a condominium in Florida and a handsome, gray-haired woman gets on with me. I notice that around her neck she wears a gold charm on a chain. It reads: "10½." I smile as I get off, wondering what friend or lover or husband had the good taste to compliment her with the gift and to recognize that she certainly is *more experienced* than Bo Derek!

In the pages of *Vogue* magazine not too many years ago, I saw a photograph of one of my favorite people, a nun by the name of Sister Serena, with whom I had once produced a touching and effective documentary film about retarded children. Standing there in the photograph, probably 60 years old at the time, with her dignity, her sense of wisdom, her elegant and beautifully expressive hands clasped before her, she makes the models who adorn the pages of the rest of the magazine look vapid and insignificant by comparison. How very beautiful she looked!

The poet Robert Penn Warren tells an interviewer, "A young man's ambition is to get along in the world and make a place for himself— half your life goes that way, till you're 40 or 50. Then, if you're lucky, you make terms with life, you get released."

"You are emancipated; you no longer have the pressures," a 54-year-old woman student at a university tells me. "You have a chance to really explore where you have never been before. You have a freedom!"

Finally, we have earned the right to our emotions, to our opinions, to our freedoms. Suddenly, we can even be *imperfect!* Some of our frustrations go back as far as our childhood, and suddenly, suddenly we find we are free. A woman of 60 recounts to me, "I had a mother who was very strict. I didn't know what it was to play with the neighborhood children, or to go out. . . . [I was] always in the house praying or going to church. So now it's time to go out and enjoy myself and to make the best of these years of my life."

For so many of us the "good old days" are, indeed, *now.* Over and over again I discover how true this is. I read the letters from my friends and the printed comments in newspapers that seem to repeat the same theme of liberation: "I have time . . ." Now there is time to try so many of the things we've postponed, and for each of us it is a different need, a different goal; we march to a different drummer, each of us, without the tyranny of ambition that colored our youthful lives.

We are at an age where we are more in touch with ourselves and with our feelings and with our needs than at any other time in our growth. And we are at an age where the dreams of our years are finally within our reach.

There is a primitive society in Southern Africa—the !Kung San—

that forbids young adults to eat the eggs of the ostrich, believing that it will make them insane. It is a special treat reserved only for very young children and for people of middle age, an unwritten link of kinship between the first generation and the last. Only when the adult has entered the middle years can he or she savor the taste of what has been withheld for generations. Then, and only then, are they allowed to eat the ostrich eggs. *We* have reached that stage in life. We need not rush through it. We can finally enjoy our own ostrich eggs, for which we have worked so hard. How marvelous that the "me" generation is finally "us."

Since so much seems to happen to me on the buses of New York, what occurred this week was no exception. Three days ago, an elderly messenger climbed aboard the Third Avenue bus. He was about 75 years of age, and as he made his way down the aisle of the bouncing vehicle, his thin, flat package clutched under his arm, he let the entire gathering of passengers know his very valid philosophy and I laughed along with the rest. "Live each day as it comes," he proclaimed loudly. "Stop looking for tomorrow. *This afternoon* ain't here yet, and you're lookin' for tomorrow!"

It is, indeed, today that matters. It is now, and for some the eating of the ostrich eggs will take the form of using the children's inheritance and setting off on a trip around the world. For others it will be a chance to change careers, to go back to school, to learn how to bake pizza, to garden—or to just sit. "For age is opportunity no less than youth itself," Henry Wadsworth Longfellow wrote. For each of us, no matter what our choosing at this stage in our lives, the opportunity will be personal and it will be rewarding.

Yes, I shall miss these friends that I've made over this past year or more, though I have tried to communicate their deep wisdom, their vitality and zest for life, and their very real awareness of themselves as people who are entering the most exciting time of their growth. I have learned much about them, but I have also learned so much about myself from them.

And for me? What will there be in these new discoveries, in this new awareness? Certainly, I hope there will be more books, and certainly, the production of the documentary films I love so much—especially those that deal with the fascinating lives of the people in the world of ours.

But what of now? What of this moment of time in my middle years, when I have just turned 58 and there are such deep feelings of joy mixed with weary achievement, and feelings of disbelief that I have reached the end of a book that I have so loved writing.

For now, I turn to a quotation that I used in a book that my wife and I wrote a few years back, little thinking then that what *began* the philosophy of one book would *end* another on exactly the right note. For now, only for this moment in time in my journey through middle life, I turn to a quotation from Thoreau and it is the last one I shall burden you with:

*Everyone should believe in something. I believe I'll go fishing.*

# Index